# Gluten-Free Cooking

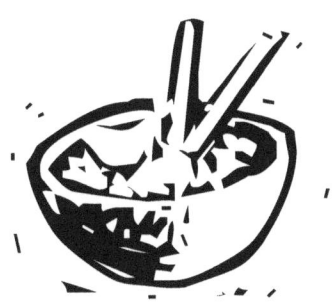

Sarah & George Holroyd

Gluten-Free Cooking

Copyright © 2023 by Sarah E. Holroyd and George E. Holroyd III
Photos copyright © 2023 by George E. Holroyd III and Sarah E. Holroyd except the mortar and pestle on page 1 and the bamboo utensils and Dutch ovens on page 2, which are used under Creative Commons licensing

ISBN: 978-0-9971590-9-7

Interior and cover design by Sarah E. Holroyd (https://sleepingcatbooks.com)

NOTICE OF RIGHTS
All rights reserved. No part of this book may be reproduced or transmitted in any form by any means (electronic, mechanical, photocopying, recording, or otherwise) without the prior written permission of the authors.

NOTICE OF LIABILITY
The information in this book is distributed on an "As Is" basis, without warranty. The authors shall have no liability to any person or entity with respect to any loss or damage caused or alleged to be caused directly or indirectly by the instructions contained in this book.

TRADEMARKS
All product names identified throughout this book are used in editorial fashion only and for the benefit of such companies with no intention of infringement of the trademark. No such use, or the use of any trade name, is intended to convey affiliation with this book.

# Contents

**Tips & Tools** ............................................. 1
**Side Dishes** ............................................. 5
    Black Beans and Rice ................................. 7
    Cornbread .................................................. 9
    Hungarian Pickled Cabbage ....................... 11
    Marinated Camembert ................................ 13
    Patatas Bravas ........................................... 15
    Roasted Potatoes and Shallots ................... 17
    Rosemary Potatoes .................................... 19
**Soups** ...................................................... 21
    Chili ............................................................ 23
    Corn Chowder ............................................ 25
    Loaded Baked Potato Soup ........................ 27
    Picadillo .................................................... 29
    Pot au Feu ................................................. 31
    White Chicken Chili ................................... 33
**Main Courses** ........................................ 35
    Broiled Tilapia .......................................... 37
    Caribbean Chicken, Chorizo, and Rice ..... 39
    Chicken Piccata ........................................ 41
    Chicken Tikka Masala ............................... 43
    Doro Wat .................................................. 45
    Glazed Salmon .......................................... 47
    Pan-fried Catfish ....................................... 49
    Red Beans and Rice .................................. 51
    Rosemary Roast Chicken .......................... 53
    Sautéed Sausage, Peppers, and Potatoes ... 55
    Sheet Pan Pork Chops ............................... 57
    Sheet Pan Tandoori Chicken ..................... 58
    Steak Maui ................................................ 61
    Taco Salad ................................................ 63
    Turmeric Chicken ..................................... 65
    Unstuffed Peppers .................................... 67
**Desserts** .................................................. 69
    Apple Tartlets ........................................... 71
    Easy Fudge ............................................... 73
    Peanut Butter Cups .................................. 75
    Rice Pudding ............................................ 77
**Index** ...................................................... 79

# Tips & Tools

### *Dried Beans*
Using dried beans is healthier than using canned beans, but takes a little more effort. Dried beans must be soaked and boiled before you can use them in a recipe. Place the beans in a saucepan and add cold water to cover the beans by several inches. Cover the pan and let the beans soak 6–8 hours, or overnight. Place the saucepan over high heat until the water begins to boil. Reduce the heat to medium and adjust as needed to keep the beans gently boiling, covered, for about an hour or until they are almost cooked (fish one out with a spoon or fork and taste-test it). **Note:** Some types of beans may take longer to cook than others. Check the package instructions. Drain the beans in a colander, allow them to cool, and store them in a sealed container until you're ready to use them.

### *Fresh Herbs & Vegetables*
To help fresh herbs, bagged salads, and fresh ginger last longer, roll them up loosely in a couple of paper towels (or place a folded paper towel in the salad bag) and put them in a plastic bag in the veggie drawer of your refrigerator. If they are in there for more than two or three days, check them and remove any wilting parts, then roll in fresh paper towels.

### *Fresh Ginger*
To easily peel fresh ginger, use the edge of a sharp spoon.

### *Mortar & Pestle*
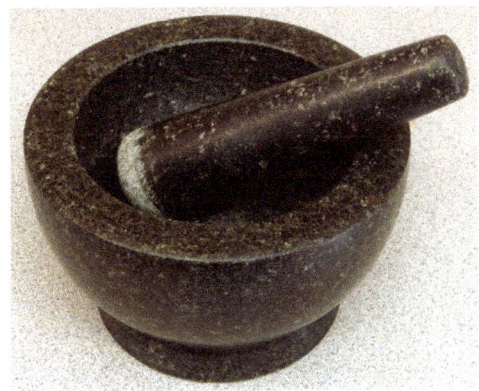
A good stone mortar and pestle comes in handy in the kitchen for grinding seeds, dried herbs, pepper corns, etc. and for creating garlic paste (*Patatas Bravas*, 15) and fresh pesto. In many applications, they can be used in place of an electric food processor.

### *Kitchen Knives*
Most kitchens need just three knives: a chef's knife (8–10" blade), a paring knife, and a bread knife. You should also have a knife sharpener. A sharp knife is far safer to use than a dull one, which can catch, skip, or slide on the food you're trying to cut and cut you! A strong pair of kitchen shears is essential as well.

# Tips & Tools

Along with knives, you will of course need at least one cutting board, although it's a good idea to have separate cutting boards for vegetables and for raw meets. Bamboo or maple are common woods for cutting boards, while dishwasher-safe plastic is good for raw meats. If you have a wooden board, consider getting a bottle of food-safe mineral oil to occasionally rub into it. This will help extend its life. Many housewares stores carry mineral oil specifically for cutting boards.

### Bamboo Utensils
A set of sturdy bamboo utensils is a good addition to your kitchen, expecially flat-edged "spatula" type ones.

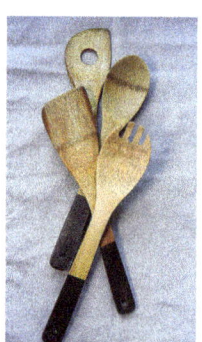

### Cheesecloth
Cheesecloth, either as a flat sheet or sewn into a small drawstring bag, is handy for containing ingredients that you'll later fish out and exclude from the final dish, such as the bouquet garni in *Pot au Feu* (31).

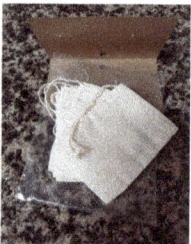

### Baking Twine or Oven-safe Elastic
This is handy for trussing a chicken, such as for *Rosemary Roast Chicken* (53).

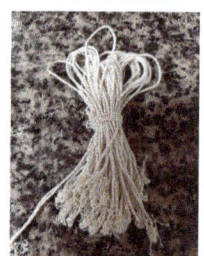

### Cooking Vessels

*Dutch Oven*

A Dutch oven is a thick-walled cooking pot that is useful for making stews. The easiest type to use and care for is enameled cast iron, such as Le Creuset or Lodge produce. For the recipes in this book, a 4.5-quart Dutch oven is a good size.

*13-inch Skillet*

Some recipes in this book, such as *Red Beans and Rice* (51), can be made in a stock pot, but they will cook more evenly (and slightly faster) if done in a large 13-inch skillet with a lid.

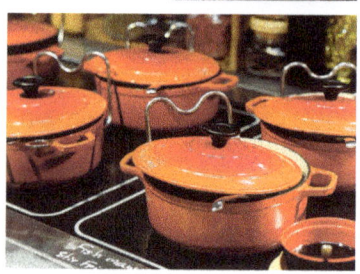

## Cast Iron Skillet

A seasoned cast iron skillet can be an invaluable addition to your kitchen. Cast iron can go from the stove to the oven and back again. This is essential for a dish like *Steak Maui* (61), which starts with a sear under the broiler, then bakes in the oven. Once the steak is cooked, the cast iron skillet goes on the stove to make a reduction sauce with the pan drippings.

## Vegetable Steamer Basket

A vegetable steamer basket makes it simple to steam fresh or frozen vegetables and retain their color and crunch. Put about 1–2 inches of water in a saucepan in which the basket will fit. Cover the pan and bring the water to a boil. Place the basket of vegetables in the saucepan, cover, reduce heat to medium, and steam for about 5–10 minutes, until desired doneness.

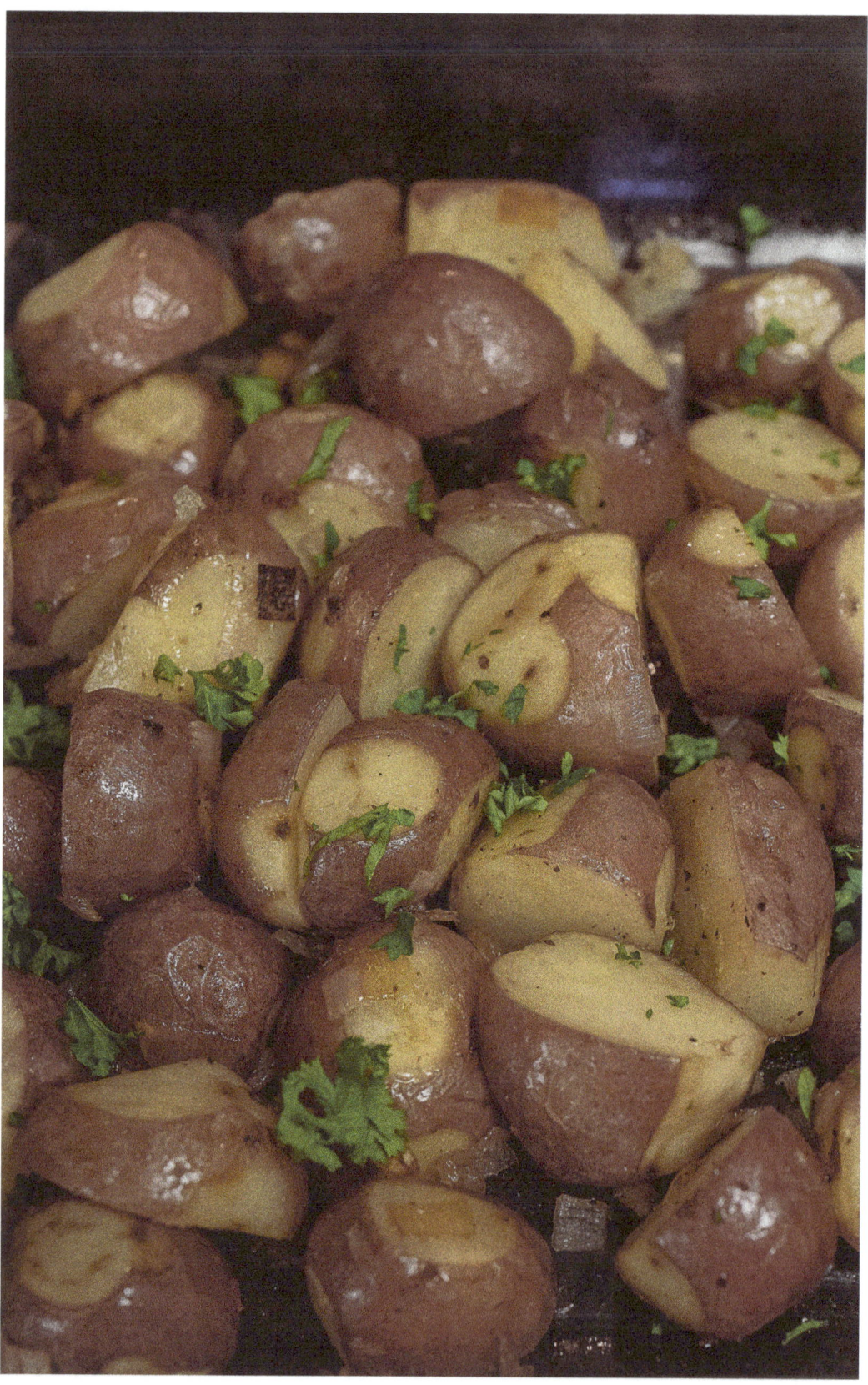

# Side Dishes

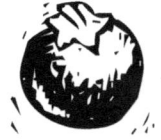

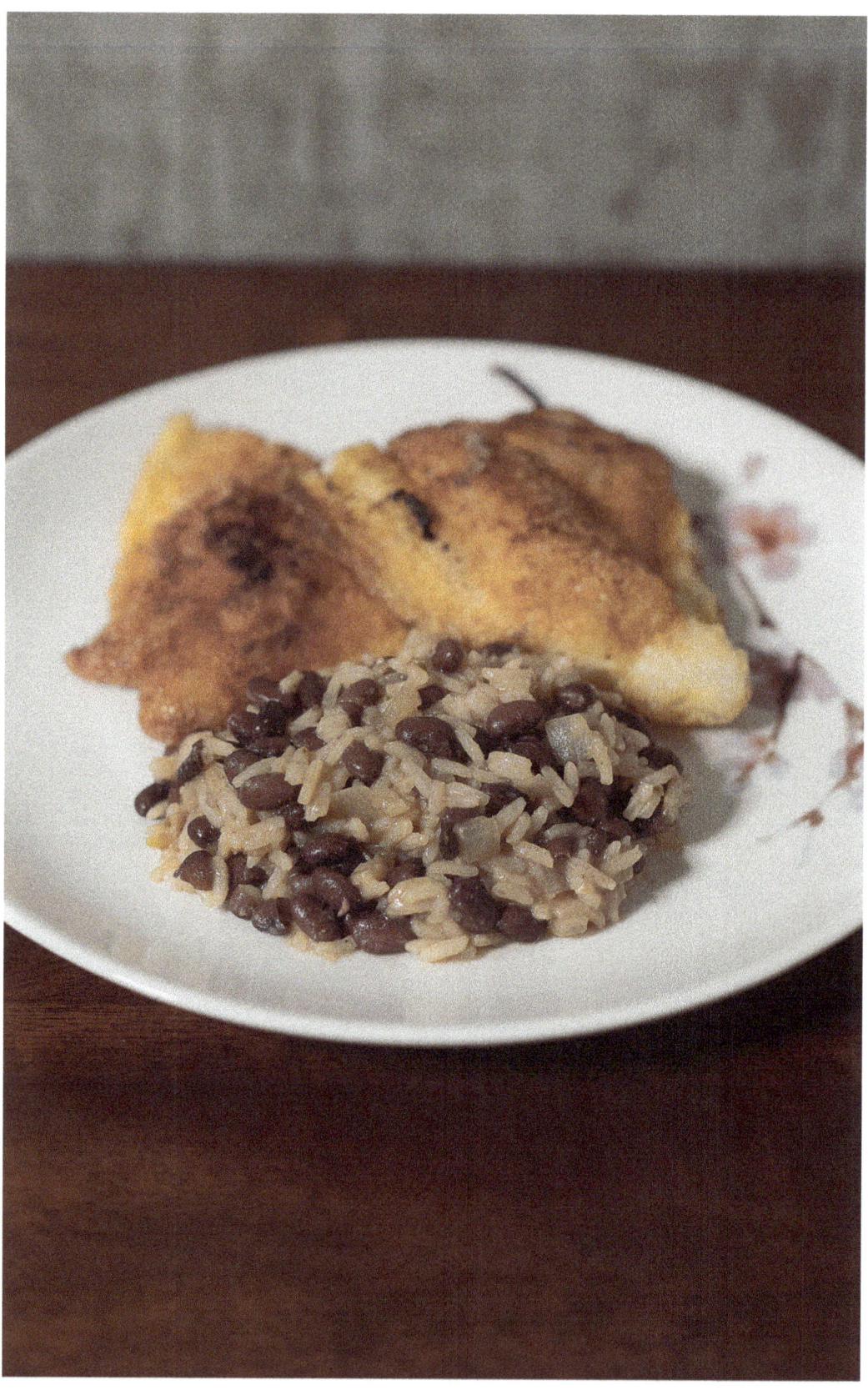

# Black Beans and Rice

1 Tbsp vegetable oil
1 small onion, chopped
1 clove garlic, minced
1/2 tsp cumin
1/2 tsp dried oregano
1/2 tsp salt*
1/8 tsp cayenne pepper
1/2 Tbsp loose brown sugar (not packed)
1/2 Tbsp white vinegar
1 1/2 Tbsp low-sodium soy sauce
1 Tbsp liquid smoke
1 15-oz can black beans, rinsed and drained (or 1/2 cup dried beans, soaked, boiled, and drained)
1 1/4 cups water
1/2 cup white rice

In a small saucepan, heat the oil over medium heat and sauté the onion and garlic until the onions begin to soften and turn translucent. Stir in the cumin, oregano, salt, cayenne, and sugar and sauté for 1 minute. Stir in the vinegar, soy sauce, liquid smoke, beans, and water and bring to a boil. Reduce heat to low, stir in the rice, cover, and simmer 15 minutes or until rice is cooked and all the water is absorbed.

*If using canned black beans, omit salt.

Makes 4 servings.

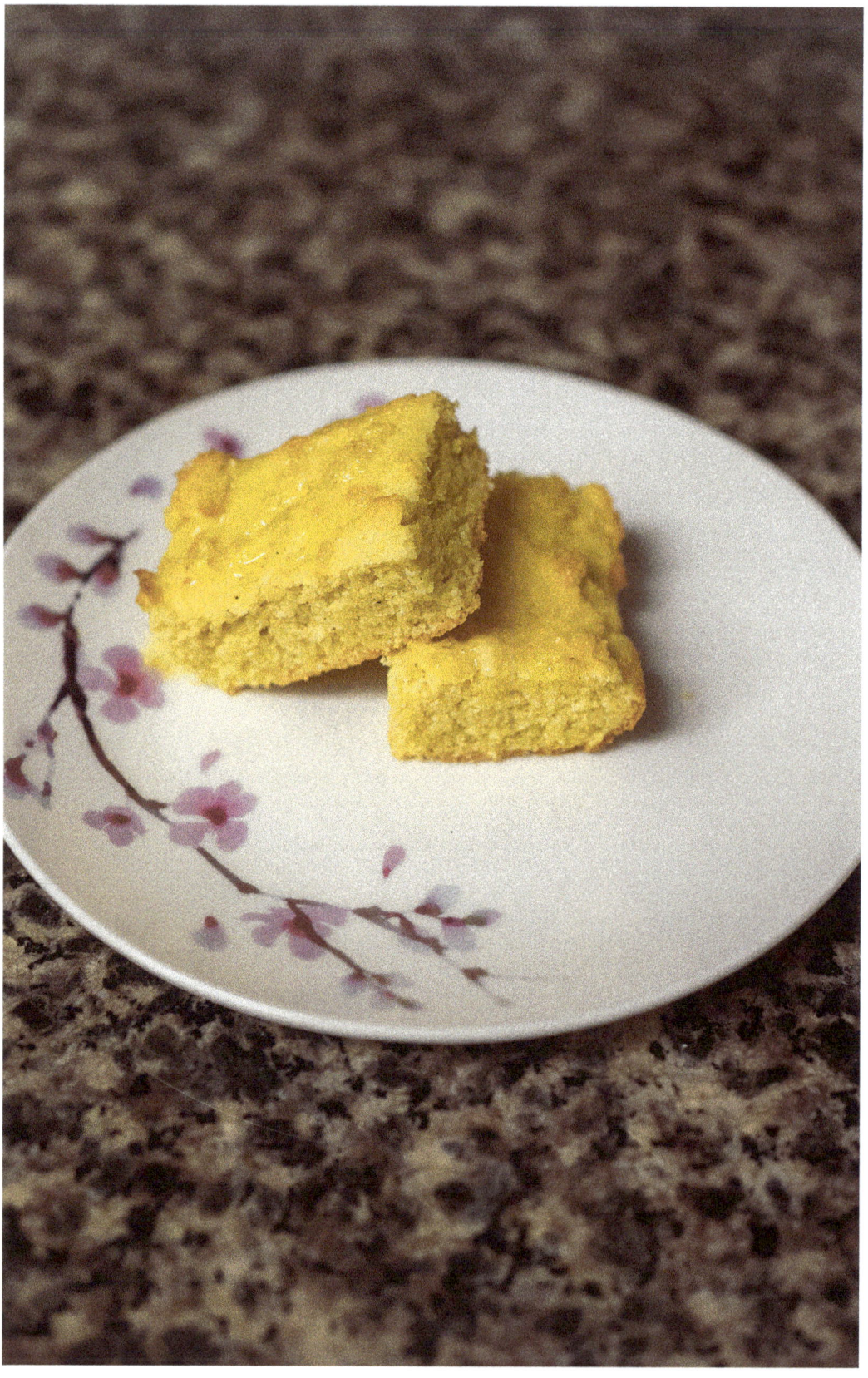

# Cornbread

butter for greasing pan
1 1/4 cups gluten-free flour*
3/4 cup corn meal
1/4 cup granulated sugar
2 tsp baking powder
1/2 tsp salt
3/4 cup milk**
1/4 cup vegetable oil
1 egg, beaten

Preheat oven to 400°F. Grease an 8- or 9-inch square pan with butter and set aside. In a medium bowl combine the dry ingredients. In a small bowl combine the milk, oil, and egg. Make a well in the center of the dry ingredients and pour the liquid ingredients in, mixing just until dry ingredients are moistened. Spread batter in prepared pan. Bake for 20–25 minutes or until light golden brown and a toothpick inserted in the center comes out clean. Cut into rectangles or squares.

*This recipe was tested with a gluten-free baking flour blend of white rice flour, brown rice flour, potato starch, tapioca flour, and xanthan gum.

**For moister corn bread, use up to 1 cup of milk.

Makes 12–16 servings.

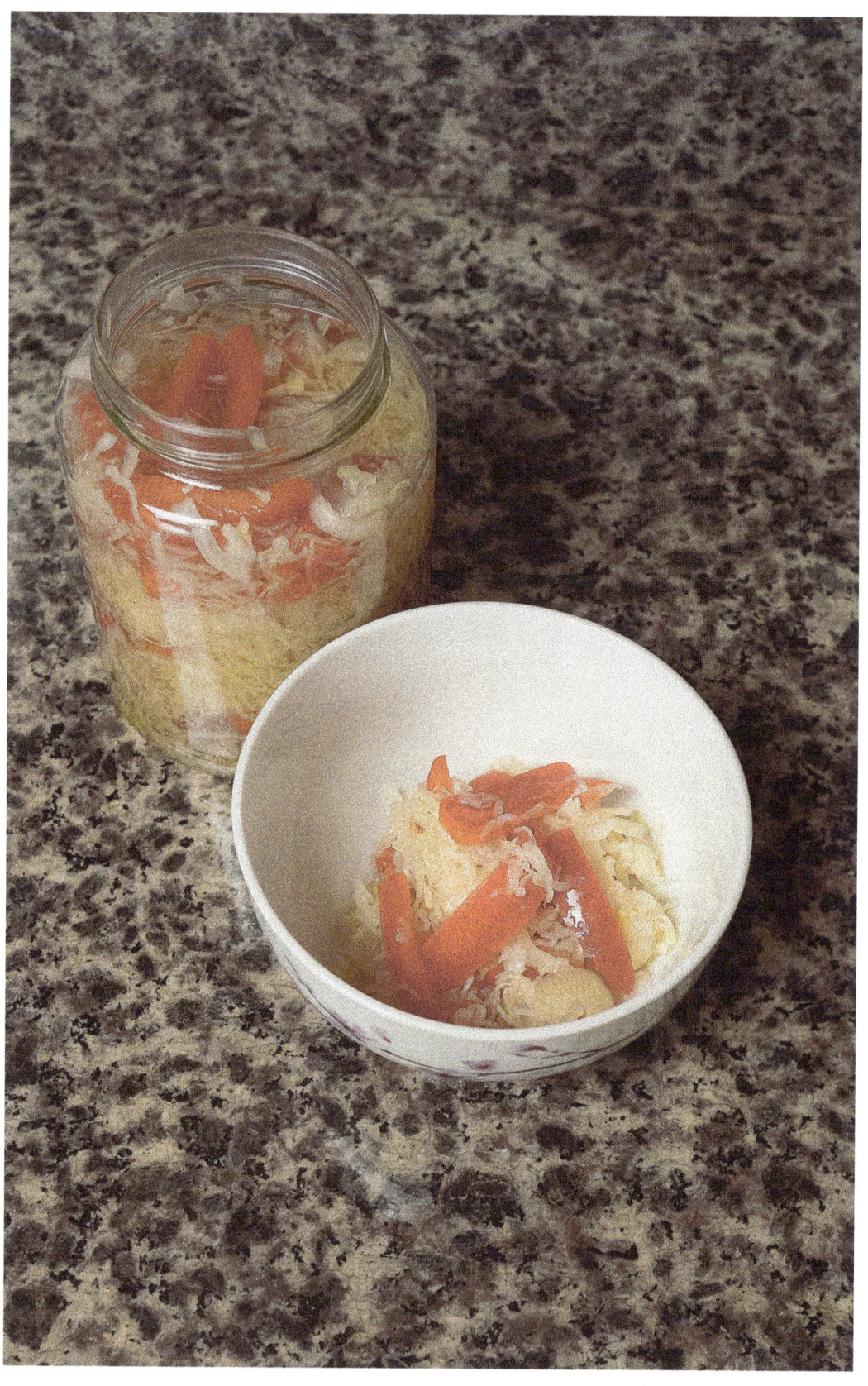

# Hungarian Pickled Cabbage

*Pickled vegetables are hugely popular in Hungary. The large Central Market in Budapest has stand after stand of tourist kitsch and jars of pickled vegetables. They would arrange the components in the jars to create smiley faces, and even landscapes!*

1 bag shredded cabbage
1 red bell pepper, quartered and sliced
1 small onion, quartered and sliced
2 1/2 tsp salt
1 1/2 cups water
1/2 cup apple cider vinegar
1/4 cup granulated sugar
1/4 tsp black pepper
1 bay leaf

In a large bowl combine the vegetables. Sprinkle the salt over and use your hands to toss. Set aside for 1 hour.

While the vegetables are standing, combine the remaining ingredients in a small saucepan and bring to a rolling boil. Remove from heat and let cool.

When the vegetables have stood for 1 hour, squeeze the excess water from them and place them in a large, clean jar. Remove the bay leaf from the liquid and pour it in the jar, seal, and refrigerate.

**Note:** If you use a cabbage mix that contains purple cabbage, the resulting pickle will take on a pink tint as it sits in the refrigerator.

Makes 6–8 servings.

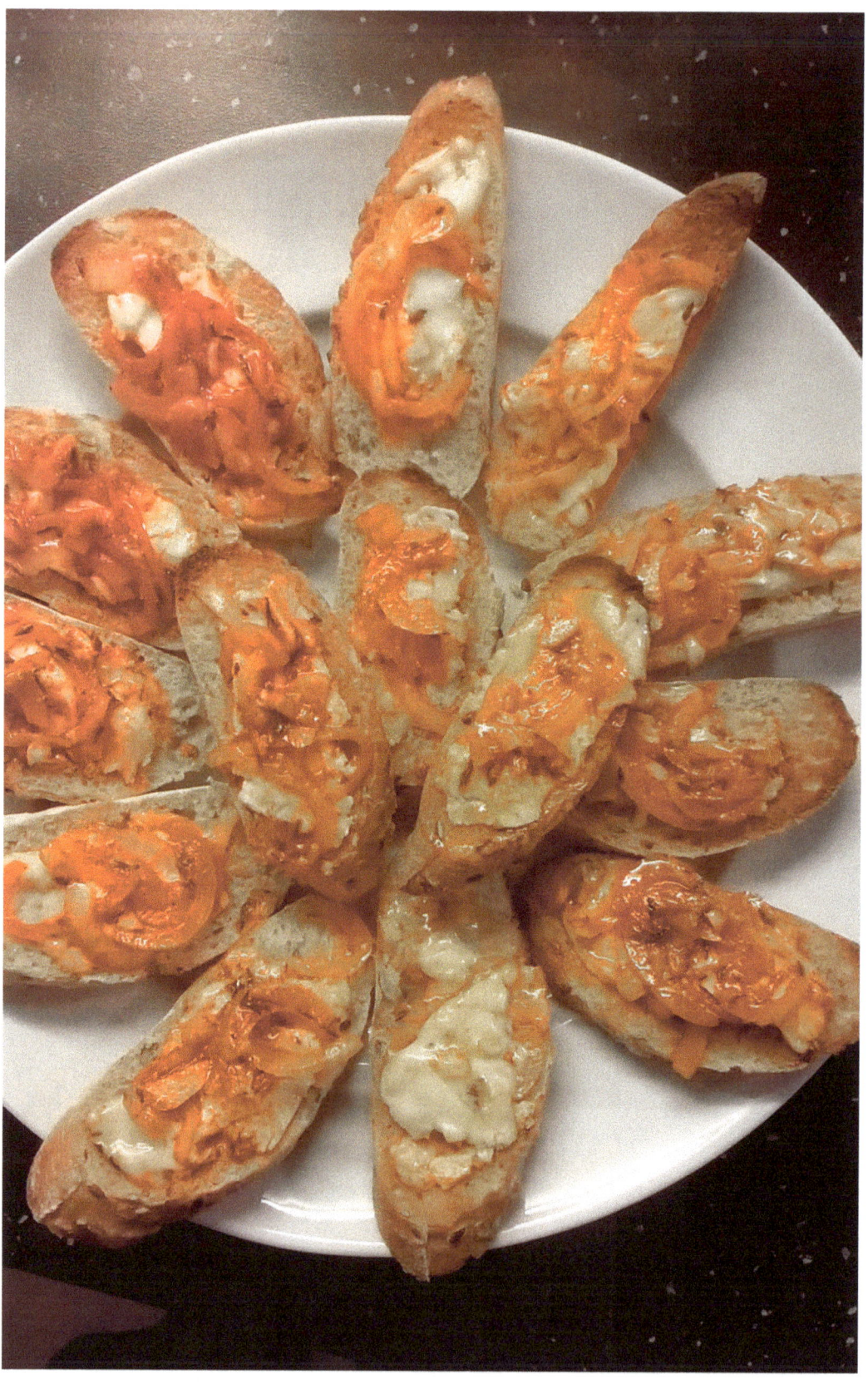

*Side Dishes*

# Marinated Camembert

*Hermelín is a Czech cheese, similar to Camembert, and is often marinated with onions, garlic, and spices. We first had it at a tiny Czech pub just around the corner from our apartment in Budapest. It makes for great pub grub spread on slices of hot toasted baguette!*

1 round block of Camembert, Brie, or Hermelín cheese
1/2 tsp cayenne pepper
1/2 Tbsp paprika
1/2 tsp dried thyme
1/4 tsp cracked black pepper
1/8 tsp salt
1 medium onion, quartered and thinly sliced
2 cloves garlic, thinly sliced
vegetable oil

Cut the cheese into 8 equal triangles and set aside.

Mix the cayenne, paprika, thyme, pepper, and salt in a large bowl. Place the cheese in the bowl and gently mix with the spices until evenly covered. Add the onions and garlic to the bowl and gently mix.

Put everything into a clean jar. Pour in enough oil to just cover everything. Gently press the cheese and onions down so everything is in the oil. Seal the jar and put in the refrigerator.

Let the cheese marinate in the fridge for at least 2 days. When taking out any cheese to eat, make sure you use a clean spoon/fork so it doesn't contaminate the rest of the cheese. Serve on your favorite toasted gluten-free bread or crackers.

Makes 8 servings.

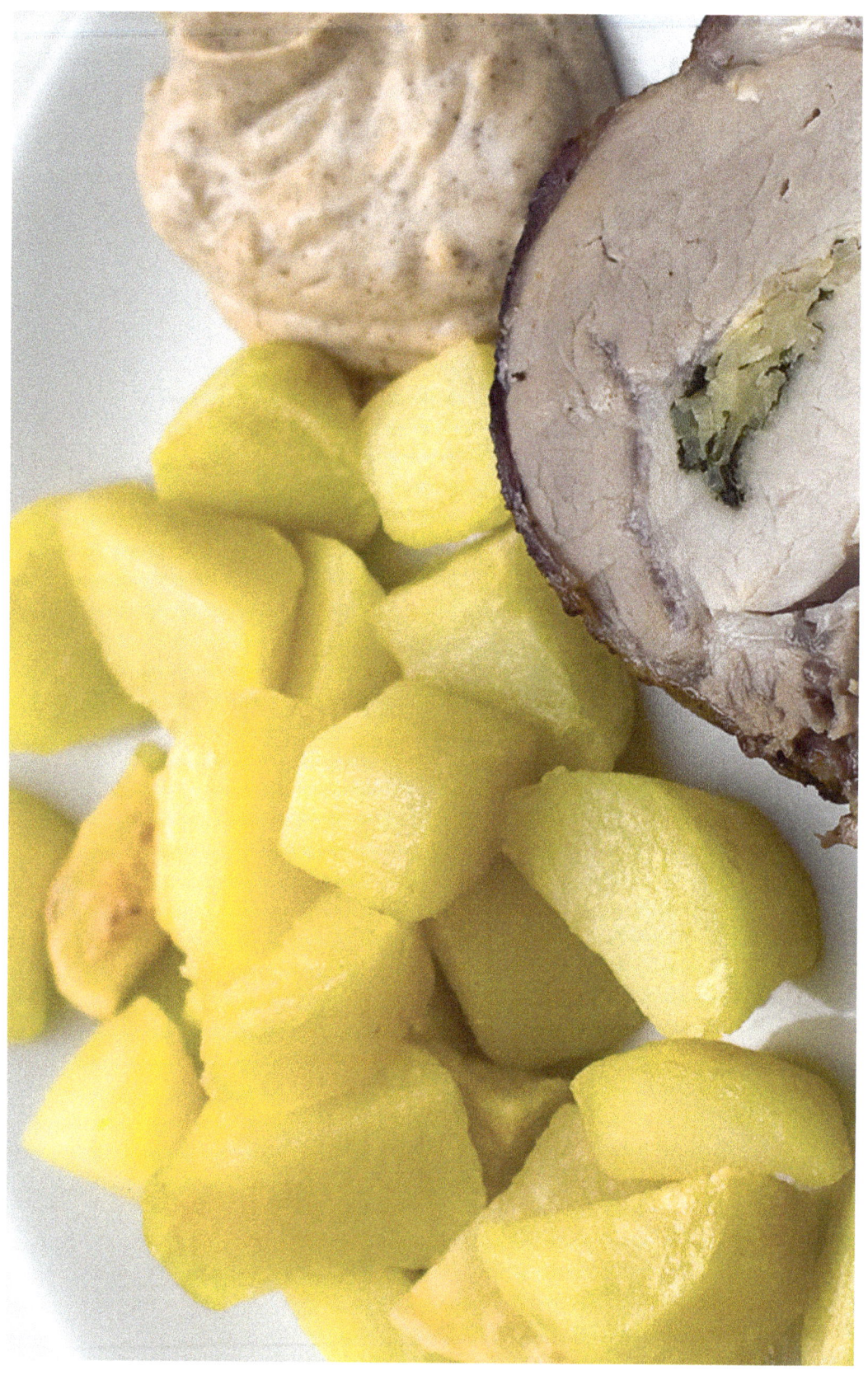

# Patatas Bravas

*We discovered this dish while on vacation in Barcelona, where you can find it at just about every tapas bar in the city. The dipping sauce with it is aioli, which is essentially garlic and mayonnaise with whatever other inclusions you wish. We made ours with lemon juice and paprika. You can either fry or bake the potatoes after blanching them in boiling water.*

1 1/2 pounds potatoes
vegetable oil

*Aioli*
2 cloves garlic, minced
1/2 tsp sea salt
1/2 cup mayonnaise
2 tsp lemon juice
1 tsp paprika

Peel the potatoes and cut into approximately 1-inch chunks. Bring water to a boil in a large pot, then add the potatoes. Boil for 5 minutes, then remove from the water. Heat about a half an inch of vegetable oil over medium-high heat in a skillet, then add the potatoes and fry until golden, turning to cook evenly. Remove to paper towels to drain off the excess oil.

While the potatoes are cooking, place the garlic and salt in a mortar and grind with a pestle to form a paste. Add several drops of lemon juice if it becomes too sticky. In a small bowl, combine the garlic paste, mayonnaise, lemon juice, and paprika until completely mixed. Taste and adjust the amounts as desired. Serve with the potatoes.

Makes 3–4 servings.

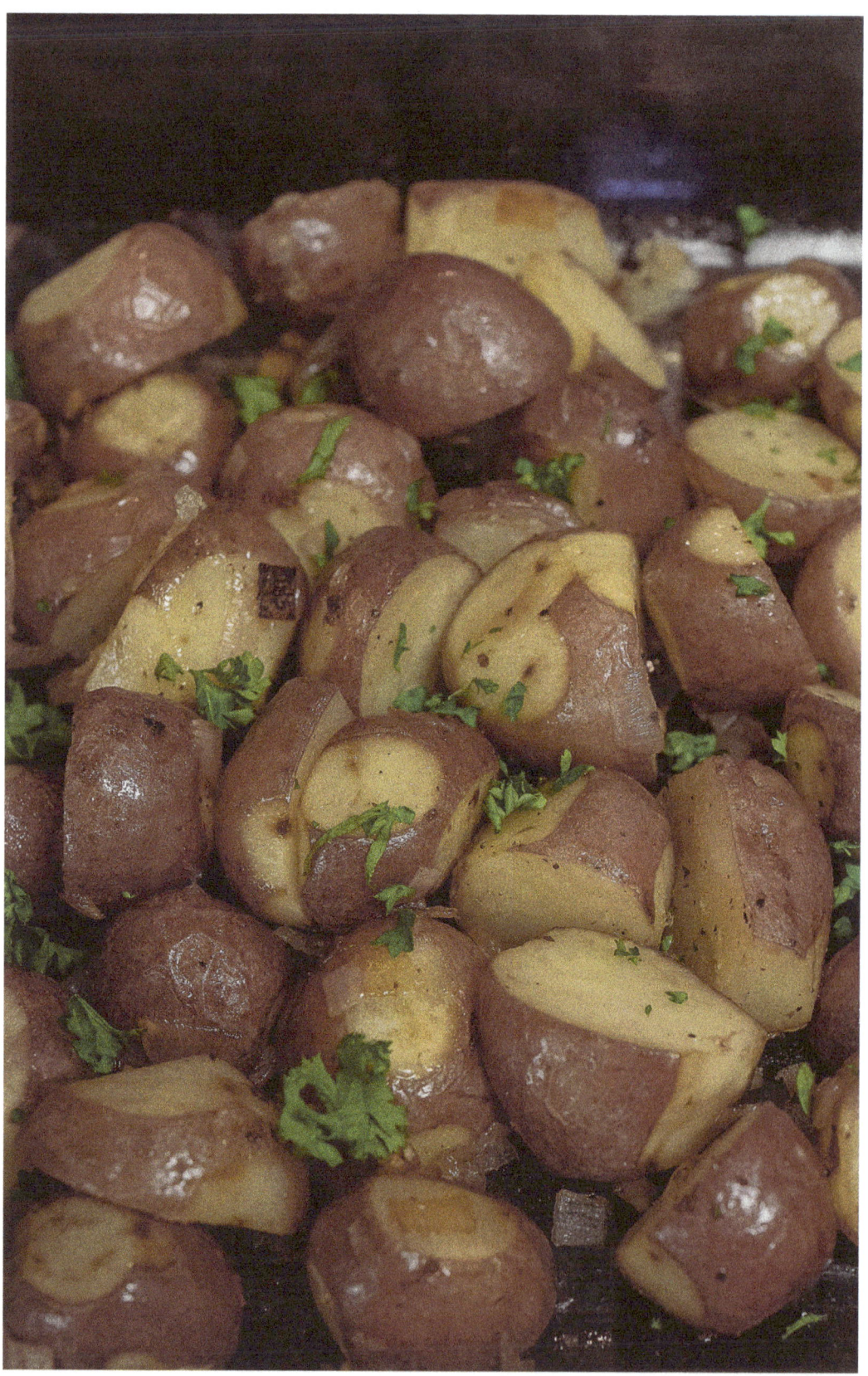

# Roasted Potatoes and Shallots

1 1/2 pounds mini red potatoes
2 large shallots
1/2 tsp sea salt
1/4 tsp cracked pepper
1 Tbsp olive oil
parsley, chopped (optional)

Preheat oven to 350°F. Wash and cut up the potatoes. Peel and coarsely chop the shallots. Mix the potatoes and shallots in a large glass baking dish with the salt, pepper, and olive oil. Bake until the potatoes are cooked through, about 30–45 minutes, stirring occasionally and adding olive oil as necessary*. Serve garnished with chopped parsley, if desired.

If you have leftover potatoes, you can use them in *Sautéed Sausage, Peppers, and Potatoes*, page 55.

*Toward the end of the cooking time they may begin to stick to the pan. Use a flat-edged bamboo stirer to scrape them up rather than adding more oil close to the end.

Makes 3–4 servings.

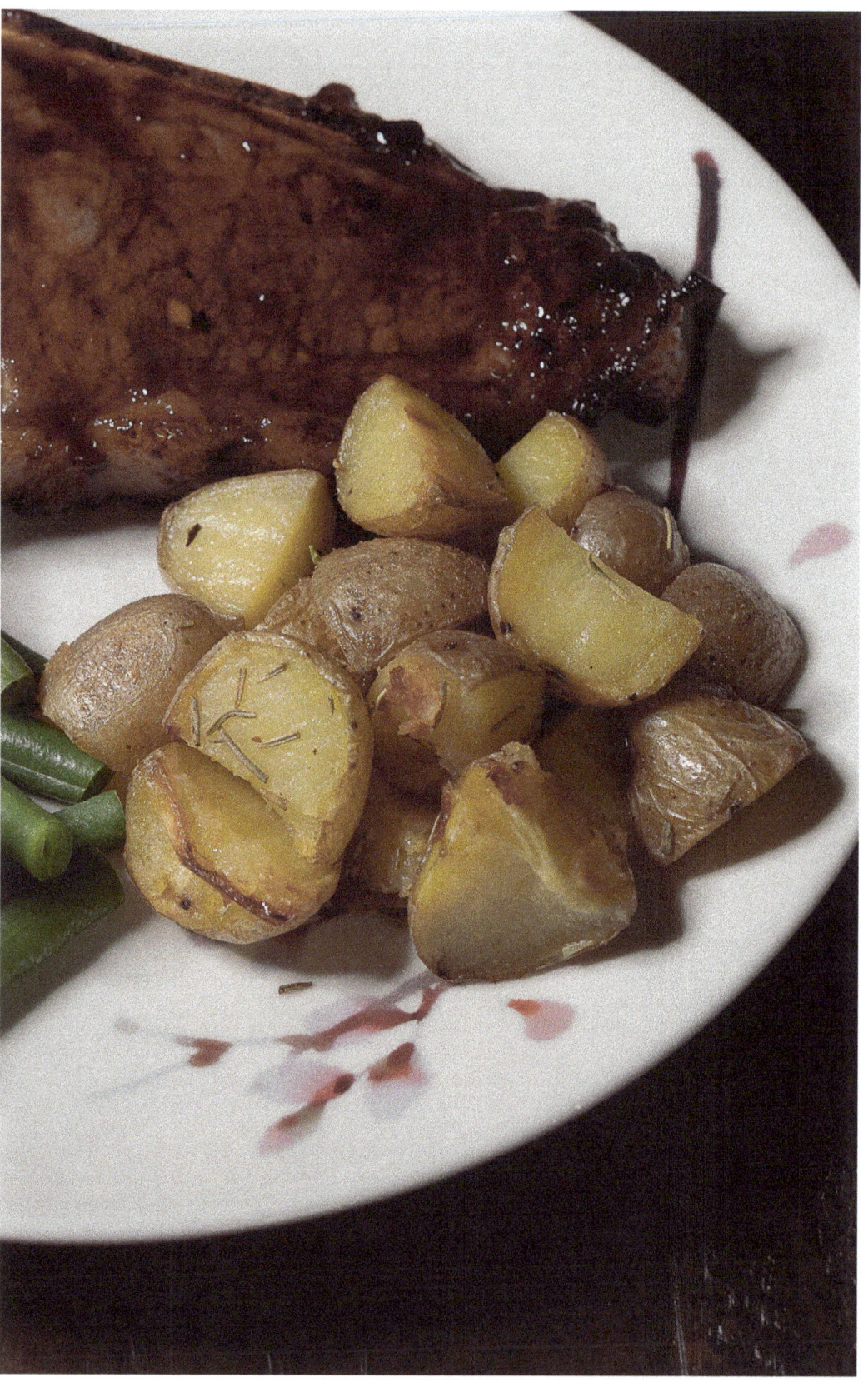

# Rosemary Potatoes

1 1/2 pounds mini gold potatoes
1 tsp dried rosemary (or 2 tsp fresh)
1/2 tsp sea salt
1/4 tsp cracked pepper
1 Tbsp olive oil
parsley, chopped (optional)

Preheat oven to 350°F. Wash and cut up the potatoes. Mix the potatoes, rosemary, salt, pepper, and olive oil in a large glass baking dish. Bake until the potatoes are cooked through, about 30–45 minutes, stirring occasionally and adding olive oil as necessary*. Serve garnished with chopped parsley, if desired.

*Toward the end of the cooking time they may begin to stick to the pan. Use a flat-edged bamboo stirer to scrape them up rather than adding more oil close to the end.

Makes 3–4 servings.

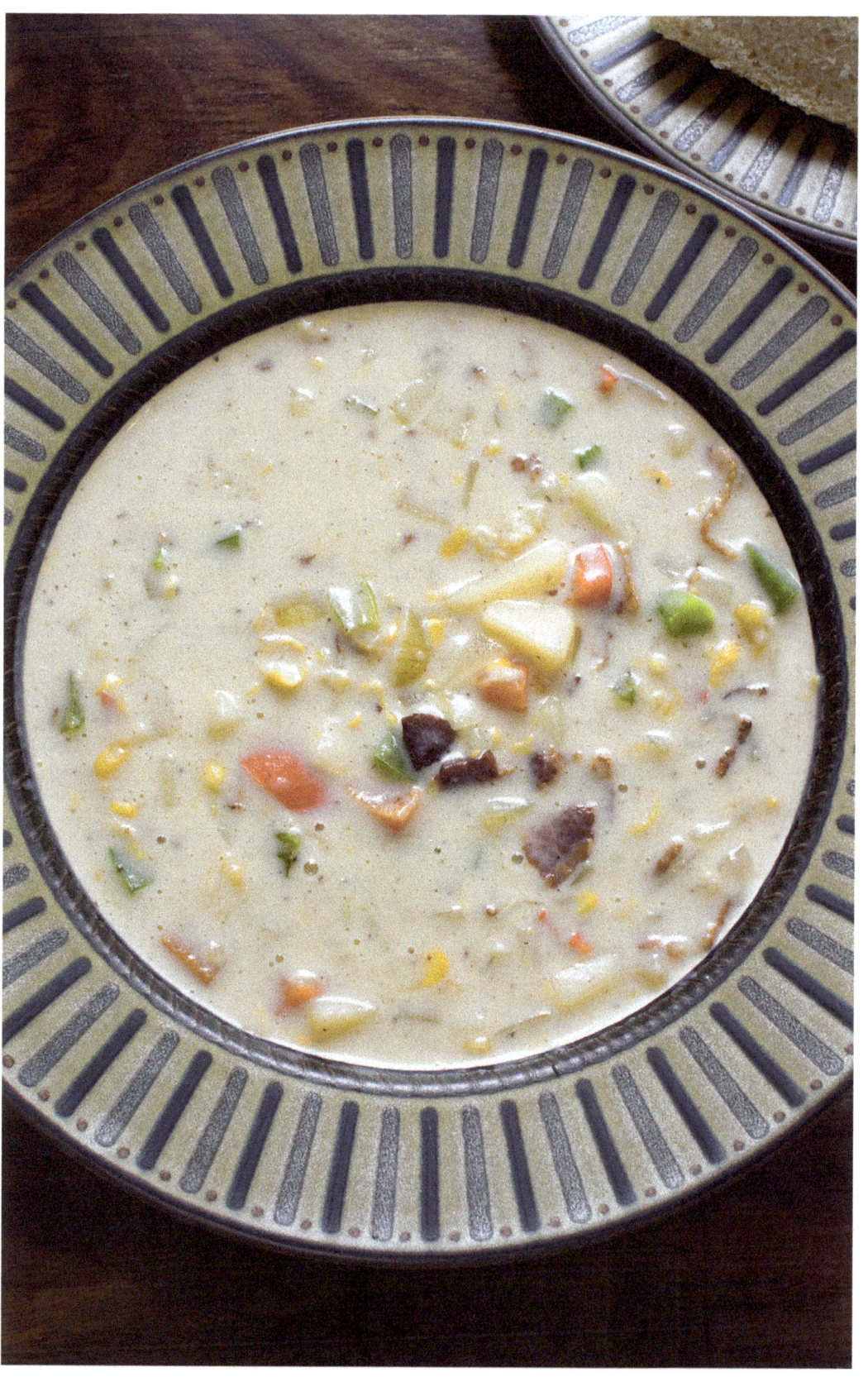

# Soups

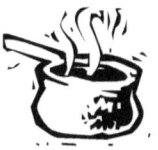

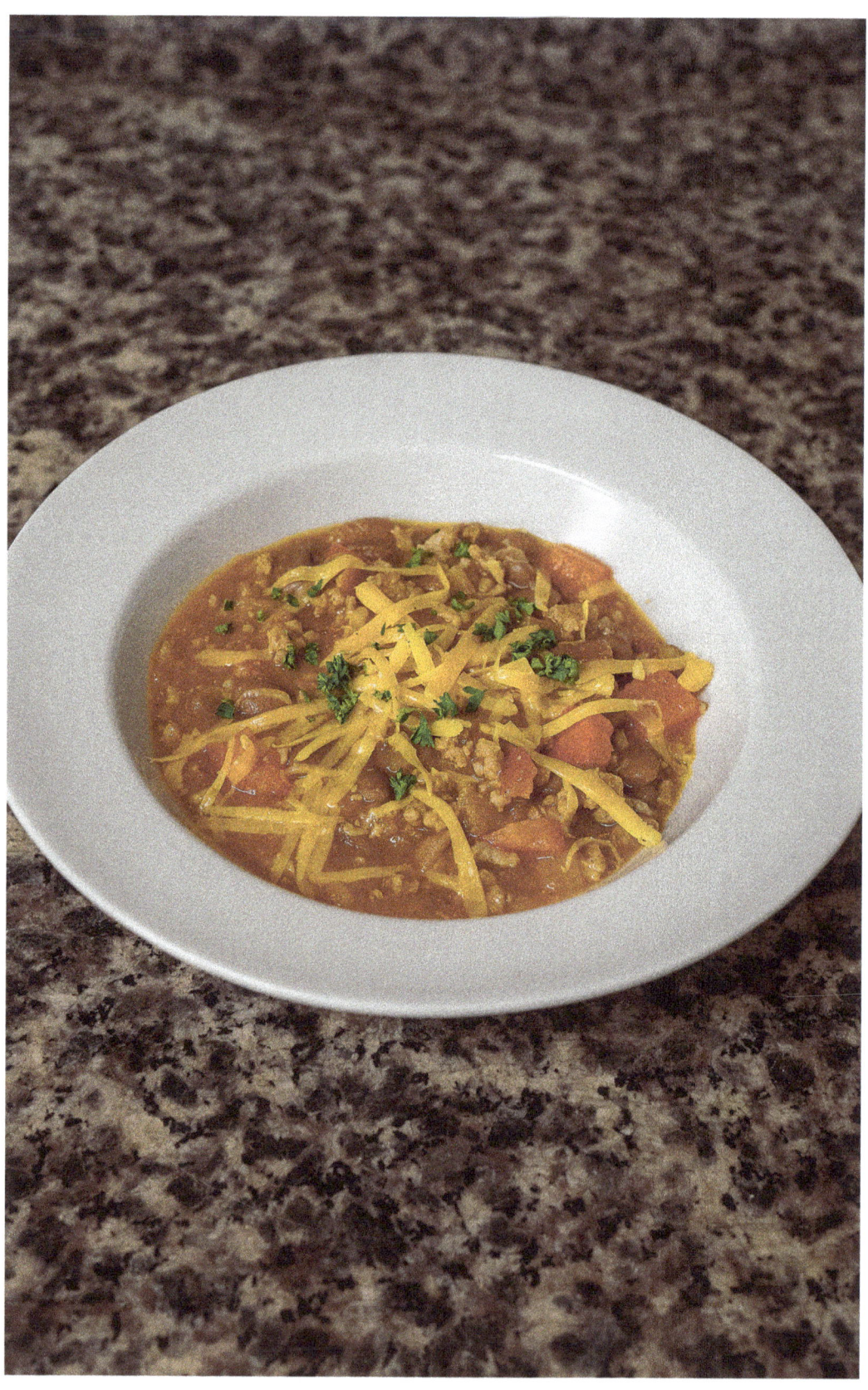

# Chili

1 Tbsp vegetable oil
1 medium onion, chopped
3 cloves garlic, minced
1 pound ground beef or pork
1 tsp cumin
3/4 tsp chili pepper
1/2 tsp salt*
1/2 tsp oregano
1/2 tsp paprika
1/4 tsp cayenne pepper
1/4 tsp black pepper
1/2 Tbsp cornstarch
2 cups water
1 red bell pepper, chopped
4 medium tomatoes, chopped
2 cans red beans, rinsed & drained (or 1 cup dried beans, soaked, boiled, and drained)
2 Tbsp double-concentrated tomato paste

In a large stock pot heat the oil over medium-low heat. Sauté the onion and garlic in the oil until the onions are translucent and begin to soften. Turn the heat to medium, add the ground meat, and brown, breaking it up as it cooks. Stir in the spices and sauté for 1 minute. Whisk the cornstarch into the water until smooth then stir into the pot, along with the remaining ingredients. Bring to a boil, stir, reduce heat to low, and simmer 45–60 minutes until thickened, stirring occasionally.

Serve with *Cornbread* (9).

*If using canned red beans, omit salt.

Makes 6 servings.

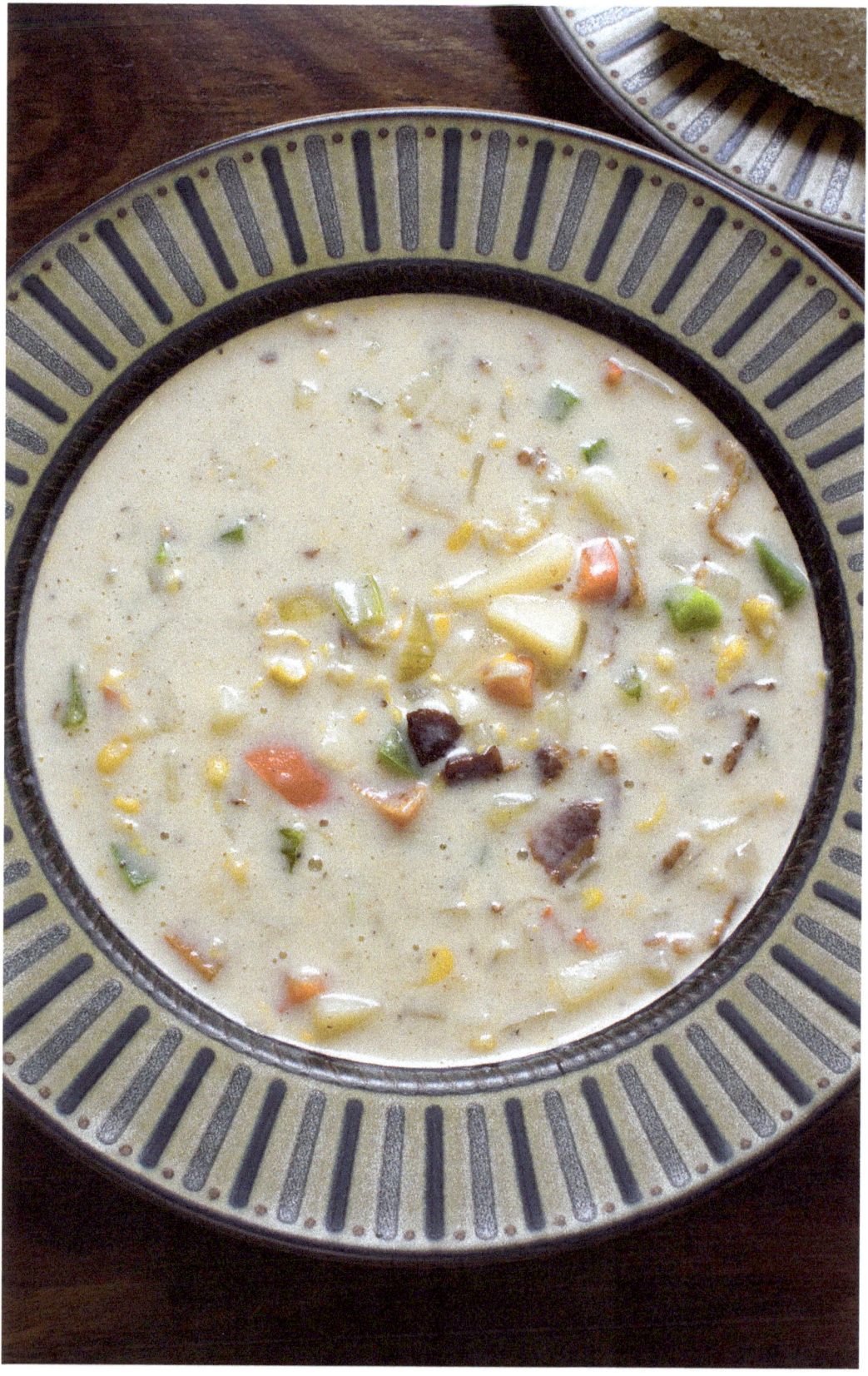

# Corn Chowder

1/2 pound bacon (about 6 thick slices)
1 medium onion, chopped
2 stalks celery, chopped
2 Tbsp cornstarch
3 1/2 cups milk, divided into 1 cup and 2 1/2 cups
1 red bell pepper, chopped
1 green bell pepper, chopped
1 14.5-oz can cream-style corn
1 14.5-oz can whole potatoes, drained & diced
black pepper to taste

Cook the bacon in a large saucepan or stock pot until crisp. Remove to paper towels to drain, then crush into bite-sized pieces. Drain the fat from the pot, leaving about 2 tablespoons. Cook the onion and celery in the bacon fat over medium-low heat until the onions are tender.

Whisk the cornstarch into 1 cup of the milk until smooth. Stir into the onions. Cook over medium heat, stirring constantly, for 1 minute. Stir in the remaining milk and the peppers. Heat to boiling, stirring constantly. Boil and stir for 1 minute. Stir in the corn, potatoes, and black pepper. Cook over medium-low heat until the soup thickens, stirring frequently. Stir in the bacon pieces and serve.

Makes 4–6 servings.

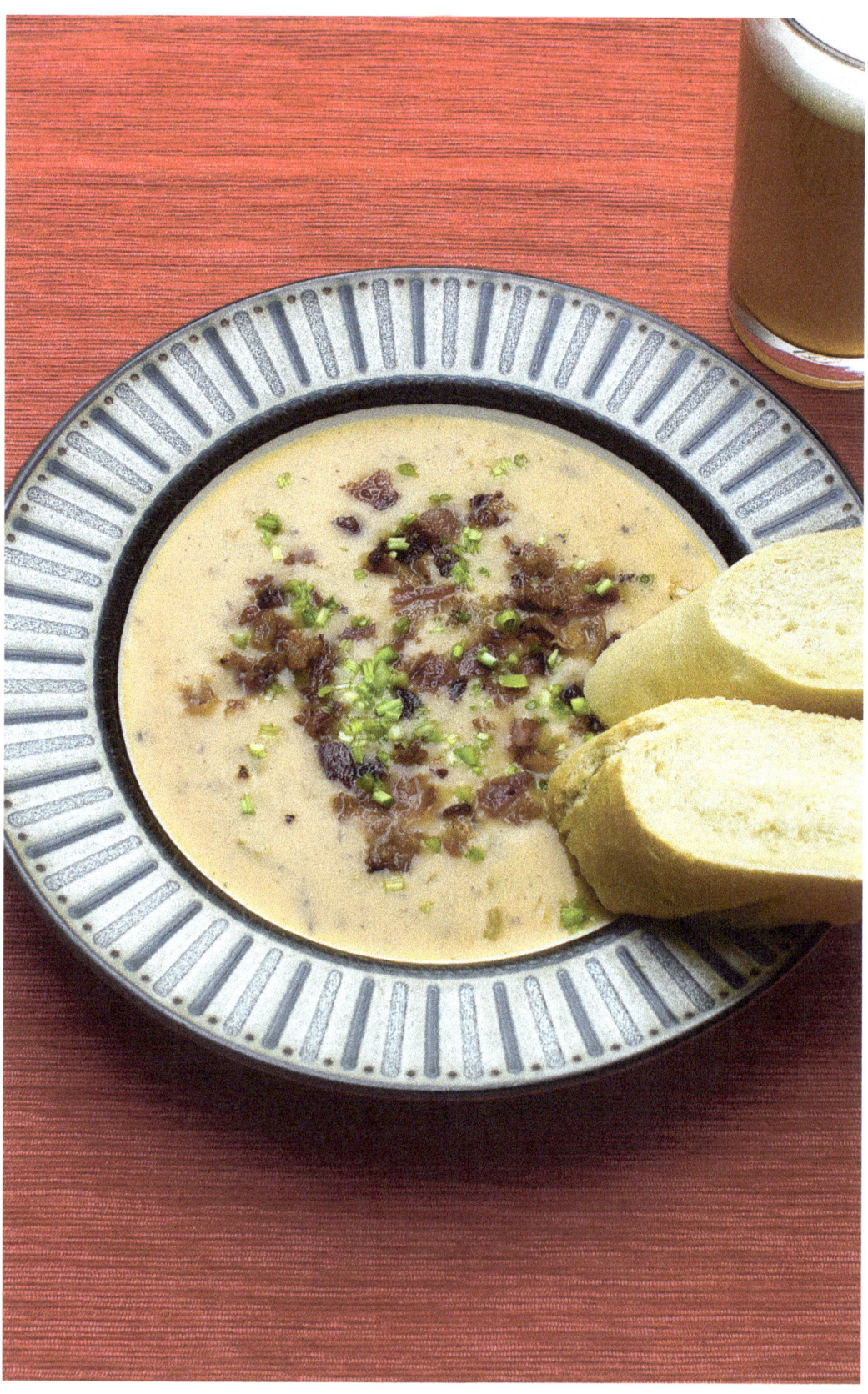

# Loaded Baked Potato Soup

6 slices thick-cut, smoky bacon
1 large onion, chopped
1 pound mini red potatoes, diced into 1/2-inch cubes (skins on)
1 Tbsp cornstarch
2 cups water
2 cups chicken broth
1/4 cup dry white wine (optional)
2 Tbsp fresh chives or green onion, chopped
sharp cheddar cheese, grated (optional)

Cook the bacon in a large, heavy saucepan or stock pot over medium heat, turning occasionally, until crisp. Transfer to paper towels to drain. Crush the bacon into bite-sized pieces; set aside. Drain fat from the pot, leaving about 2 tablespoons.

Cook the onion in the reserved bacon fat over medium-low heat, stirring occasionally, until softened and beginning to turn translucent. Whisk the cornstarch into the water until smooth, then add to the onions. Add the potatoes and chicken broth. Simmer for 10 minutes over medium heat, or until the potatoes are just tender, stirring frequently. Using a hand masher, mash some of the potatoes in the pot to help thicken the soup. If desired, add the wine and simmer 1 minute.

Serve with bacon, chives or green onion, and cheese sprinkled on the top.

Makes 4 servings.

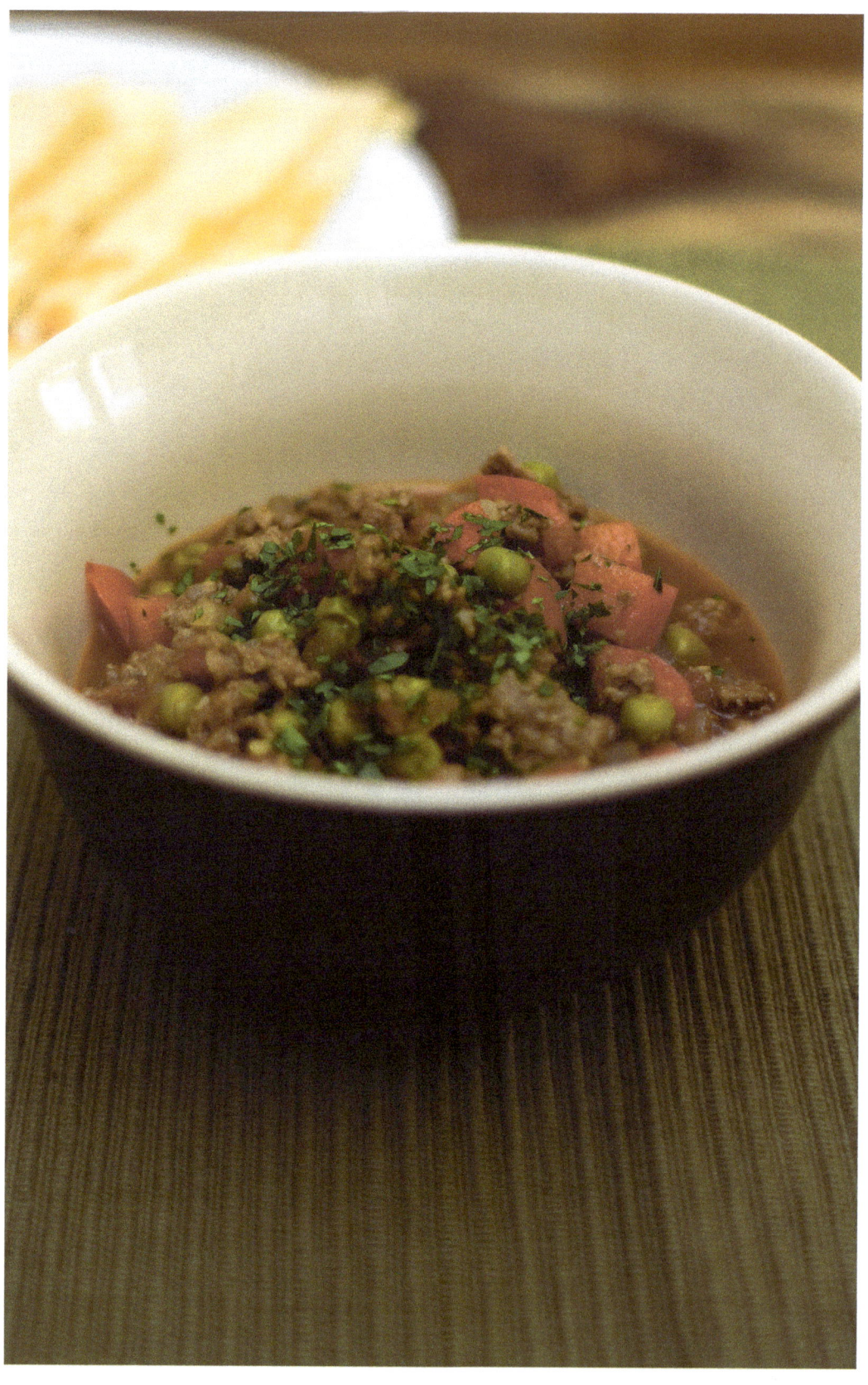

# Picadillo

1 pound ground beef or pork
1 large onion, chopped
1 red bell pepper, chopped
2 cloves garlic, minced
1 1/2 tsp cumin
1/4 tsp cayenne pepper
1 14.5–15-oz can diced tomatoes, drained
1 cup canned beef stock or broth
1/2 cup frozen peas
2 Tbsp capers, drained

Brown the ground meat in a large saucepan or stock pot over medium heat just until it is still a little pink inside; drain. Add the onions, peppers, garlic, cumin, and cayenne pepper to the pan and sauté for about 5 minutes, or until the beef is completely cooked and the onions begin to soften. Add the tomatoes, beef stock, peas, and capers. Bring to a simmer over medium heat, then reduce the heat to low and simmer, stirring occasionally, about 20 minutes.

Makes about 4 servings.

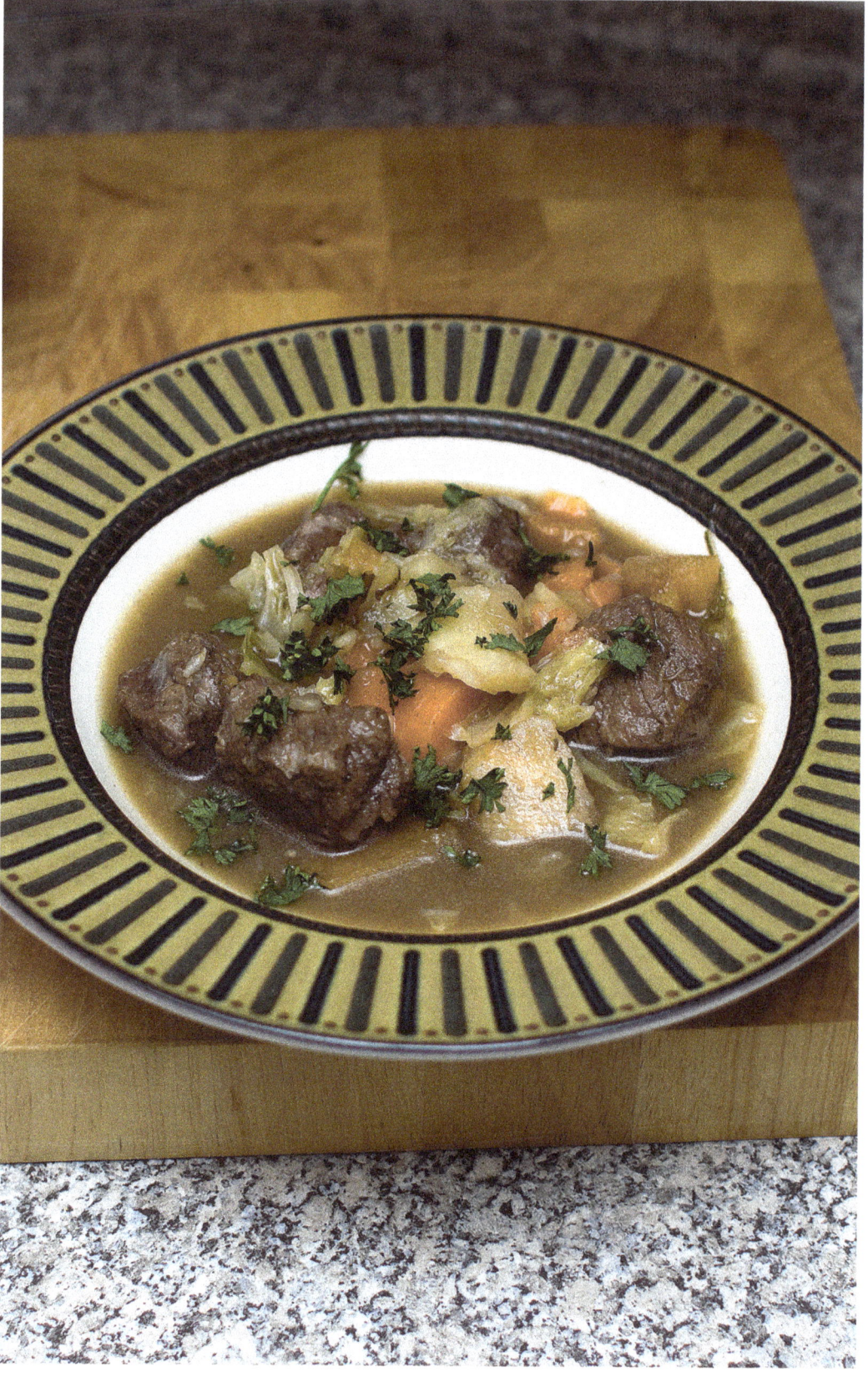

# Pot au Feu

1/4 celeriac
1/4 parsnip
1 small yellow onion
4 carrots
1 bunch fresh parsley
1 pound stewing beef or short ribs, cubed
1 Tbsp butter
1 Tbsp olive oil
3 cups water plus water to mix with cornstarch
1 cup Pinot Noir red wine
2 cups beef stock
1/4 white cabbage, chopped (optional)
1/2 Tbsp cornstarch

*Dry Rub*
2 tsp dried thyme
2 tsp dried rosemary
1 tsp kosher or sea salt
1/2 tsp cracked black pepper

*Bouquet Garni (tied in cheese cloth)*
1 bay leaf
several sprigs thyme
2 whole cloves

Rinse and coarsely chop the celeriac, parsnip, yellow onion, carrots, and parsley; set aside. Prepare the dry rub by crushing the thyme, rosemary, salt, and pepper with a mortar and pestle. Add the dry rub to the beef, turning to coat evenly. In a large stock pot, melt the butter and olive oil over medium heat. Add the beef and brown on all sides. Once browned, remove the beef to a plate and add the vegetables (except cabbage and parsley) to the pot. Lay the beef on top of the vegetables and place the bouquet garni in the center. Add the water, wine, and beef stock, cover, and bring to a boil over high heat. Reduce heat to low and simmer for 2 1/2 hours.

Add the chopped cabbage and continue to simmer for 30 minutes. Remove the beef and vegetables from the pot and strain the broth; return the broth to the pot over medium heat. Create a slurry of cornstarch and water and stir into the broth to thicken it. Bring it to a boil over medium heat, stirring constantly, and boil for 1 minute or until thickened. Remove fro heat. Place the beef and vegetables in bowls, add the broth, and garnish with chopped parsley.

Makes 4–6 servings.

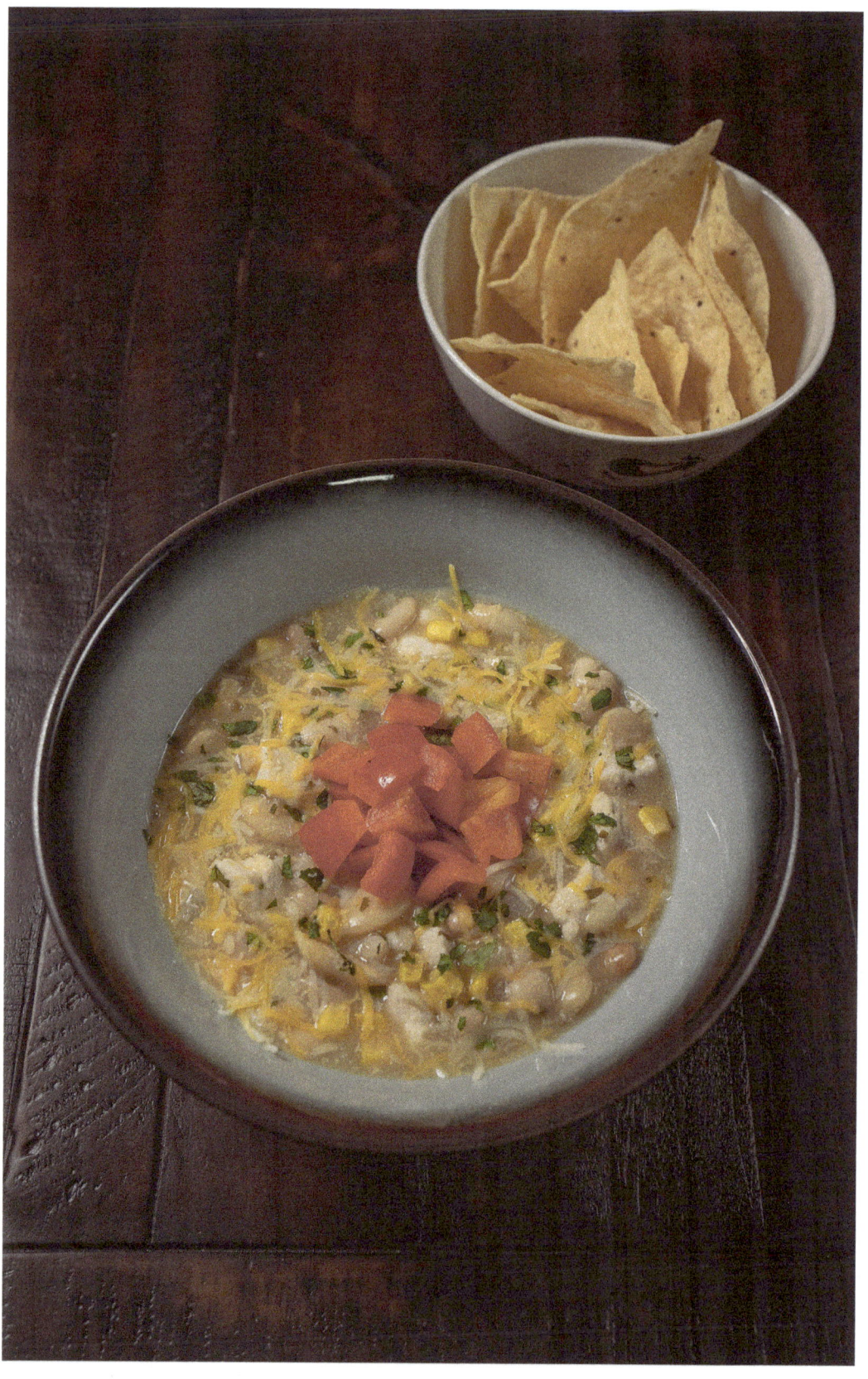

# White Chicken Chili

*A friend gave us the basis for this recipe so that we could make a double batch ahead of time and freeze it for a party. We tried some for dinner when we made it, and liked it enough to keep it in our repertoire, with some changes from the original.*

1 Tbsp vegetable oil, plus 1–2 tsp to cook chicken
6 boneless, skinless chicken tenders, diced (or 4 boneless, skinless breasts)
2 medium onions, chopped
2 cloves garlic, minced
2 Tbsp cornstarch
1 32 oz. carton low sodium chicken broth, divided into 1 cup and remainder
1/2 Tbsp dried cilantro (or 1/4 cup fresh cilantro, chopped)
2 Tbsp lime juice
1 tsp cumin
1/2 tsp dried oregano
1/2 tsp Sriracha or Tabasco sauce
1/4 tsp salt
1 can whole kernel corn, drained
2 cans great northern beans, drained
1 can butter beans, drained
toppers (shredded cheese, chopped red peppers, salsa, sour cream, etc.)

Heat 1–2 teaspoons of oil in a nonstick skillet over medium heat and cook the chicken just until it is no longer pink inside. Set aside.

Heat 1 tablespoon of oil in a large stock pot over medium-low heat. Sauté the onions and garlic until the onions are tender and translucent. Whisk the cornstarch into 1 cup of the chicken broth until smooth. Add to the onions in the stock pot with the rest of the broth. Stir in all the remaining ingredients, except the chicken. Heat to boiling, then reduce heat to low. Simmer uncovered for 20 minutes, stirring occasionally. Stir in the chicken and simmer another 10 minutes. Serve with a variety of toppers like shredded cheese, chopped red peppers, salsa, sour cream, etc.

Makes 4–6 servings.

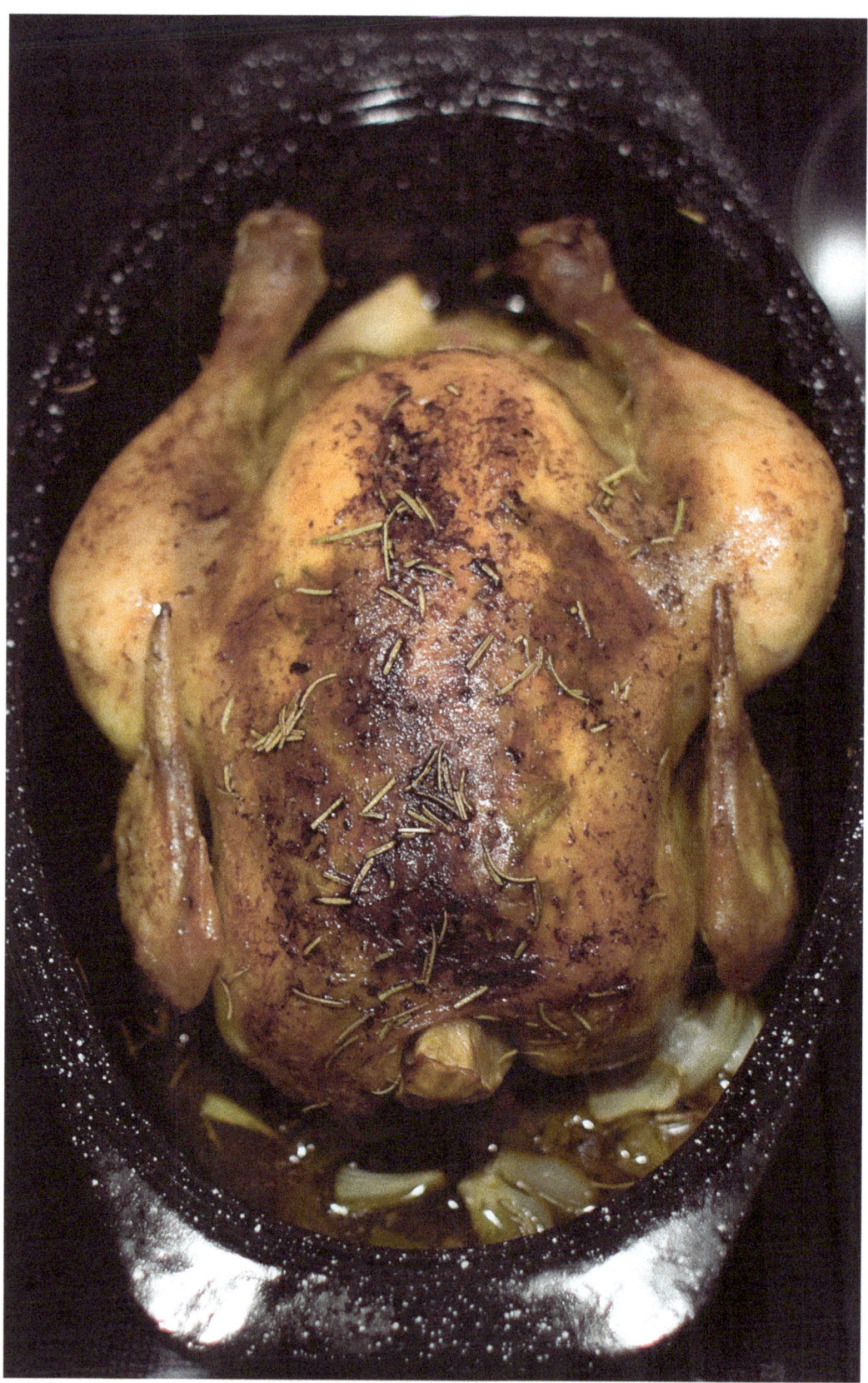

# Main Courses

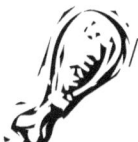

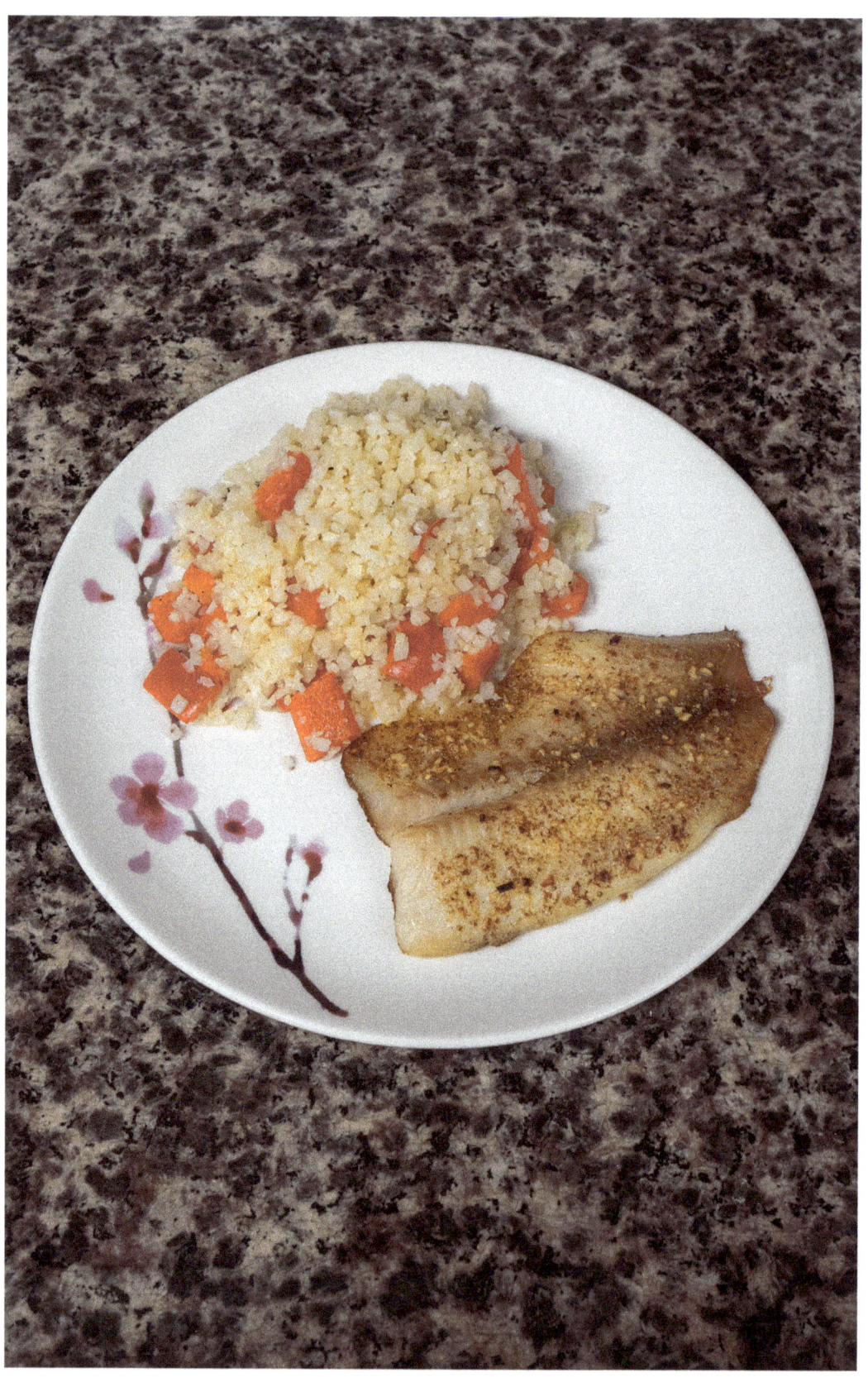

# Broiled Tilapia

*Compound Butter*
3 Tbsp butter, softened
1 Tbsp fresh basil, chopped (optional)
1/2 tsp Old Bay seasoning
1/2 tsp lemon juice
1 clove garlic, minced

2 tilapia fillets (about 1/4 pound each)
2 tsp vegetable oil (approximately)
1 red bell pepper, chopped
1 10-oz bag frozen riced cauliflower

Preheat the oven broiler with the rack at the top of the oven. Combine the compound butter ingredients in a small bowl. Set aside.

Preheat the oven broiler with the rack at the top of the oven. Place the fillets in a square glass casserole dish (like Pyrex) that is just big enough to fit them. Combine the other ingredients to form a compound butter. Spread the compound butter evenly over each fillet. Broil 5–10 minutes until the fish is translucent and flaky and the garlic pieces are golden brown.

While the fish is cooking, heat the oil over medium-low heat in a small skillet, then add the red peppers. Sauté just until they begin to soften, about 5 minutes. Remove from heat and set aside, uncovered.

Cook the cauliflower according to the package directions, then pour into a heat-resistant bowl. Add the red peppers. Remove the fillets from the casserole dish and pour the liquid from the dish into the cauliflower and peppers and mix well.

Makes 2 servings.

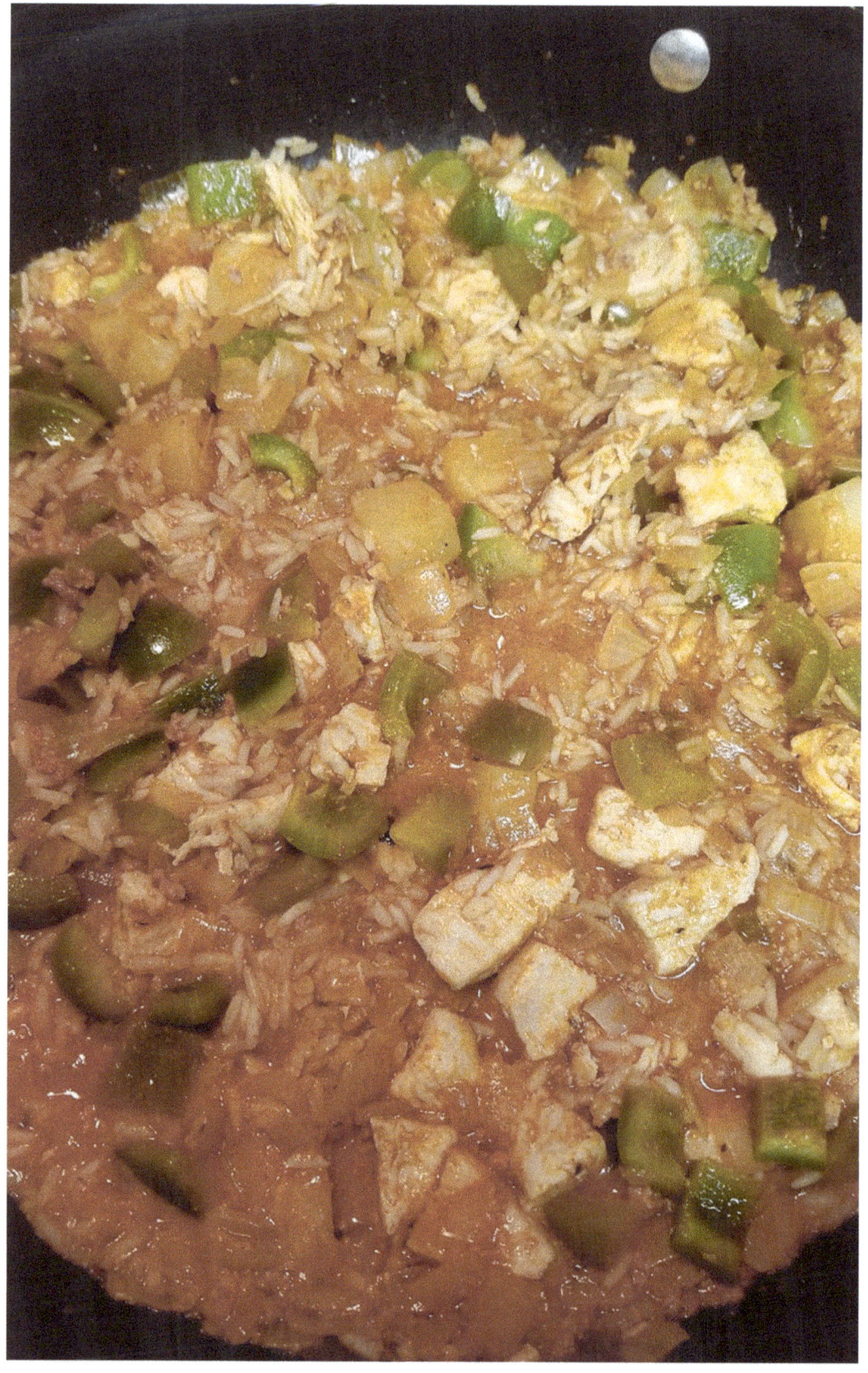

# Caribbean Chicken, Chorizo, and Rice

1–2 tsp vegetable oil

1 large boneless chicken breast or 3–4 tenders, diced

13.5 oz. gluten-free chorizo smoked sausage (Johnsonville), sliced

1 medium onion, chopped

2 cloves garlic, minced

1–2 tsp cumin

1/2 tsp oregano

1/4 tsp cayenne pepper

1 chicken bouillon cube

2 1/4 cups water

1 cup white rice

1 large green bell pepper, chopped

2 Tbsp double-concentrated tomato paste

1 cup diced pineapple, drained and further chopped

In a large skilet, heat the oil over medium heat and sauté the chicken until it is white on the outside and just cooked through. Set aside.

Sauté the chorizo until about half-way browned. Add the onion and garlic and continue sautéing until the onions begin to soften and turn translucent. Stir in the cumin, oregano, and cayenne. Add the bouillon cube, water, rice, green pepper, tomato paste, pineapple, and chicken. Bring to a boil, stir, reduce heat to low, cover, and simmer 15–20 minutes, or until all of the water is absorbed and the rice is fully cooked.

Makes 4 servings.

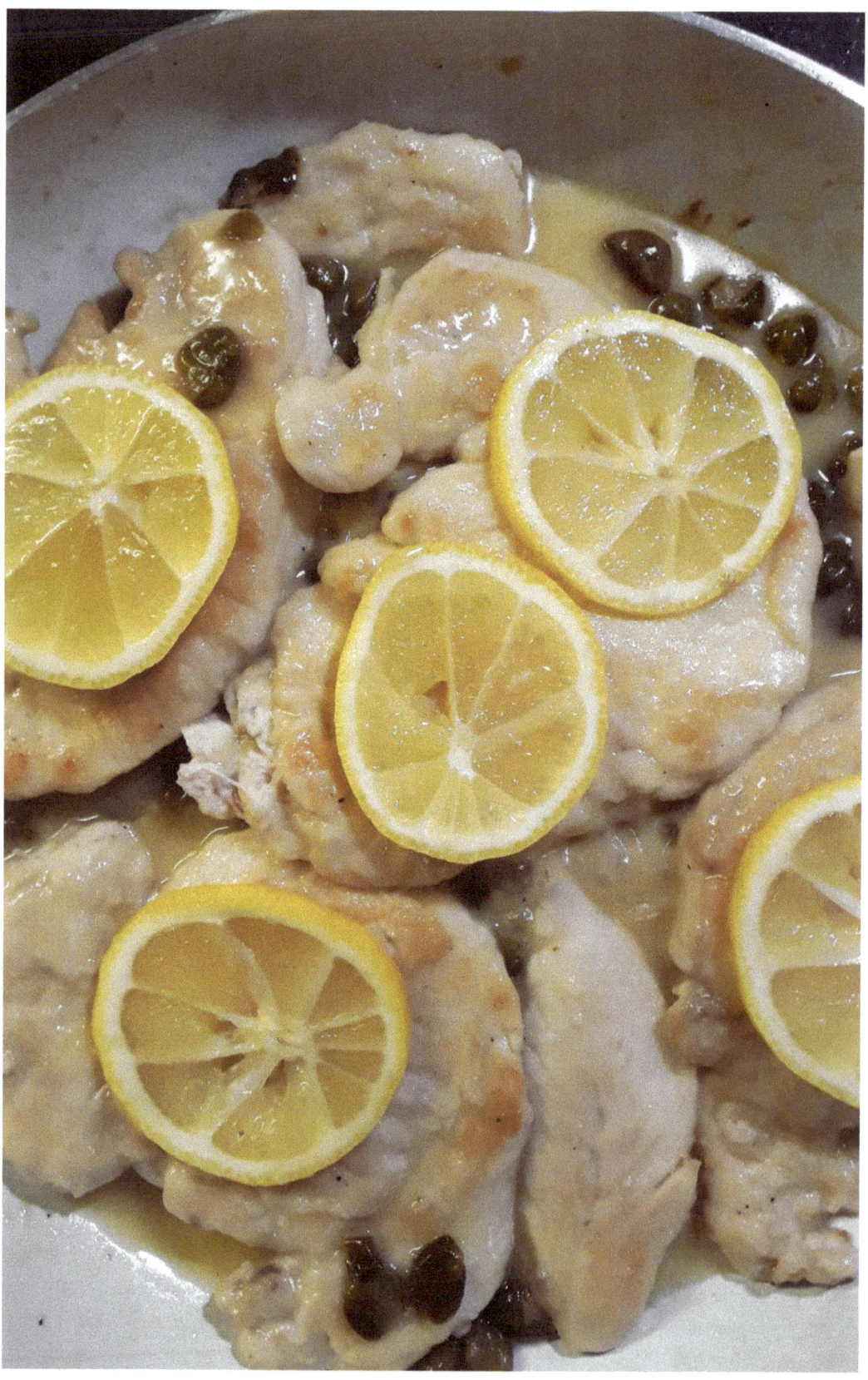

# Chicken Piccata

1 Tbsp cornstarch
1/4 cup water
2 boneless, skinless chicken breasts
1/4 cup gluten-free flour*
salt to taste
black pepper to taste
1–2 Tbsp vegetable oil
lemon slices (optional)

*Sauce*
1/2 cup dry white wine
1/2 cup chicken stock
1 Tbsp lemon juice
1/2 Tbsp butter
2 Tbsp capers, rinsed and drained

Whisk the corn starch into the water; set aside. (Whisk it again just before using it.)

Trim any excess fat or gristle from the chicken breasts and butterfly them. Pour the flour on a large plate and season with the salt and pepper. Dredge each chicken piece in the seasoned flour.

Heat the oil in a medium to large skillet over medium heat. Fry the chicken for 3 minutes on each side, then remove to a plate and tent with foil.

Add the wine, stock, and lemon juice to the skillet to deglaze it over medium heat. Add the cornstarch slurry a little at a time, stirring constantly, until the sauce thickens. You may not need all of the slurry. Stir in the butter and capers, then add the chicken pieces, turning to coat them evenly. Remove the chicken to plates and pour the sauce evenly over them. Garnish with lemon slices, if desired.

Serve with *Rosemary Potatoes* (19).

*This recipe was tested with a gluten-free baking flour blend of white rice flour, brown rice flour, potato starch, tapioca flour, and xanthan gum.

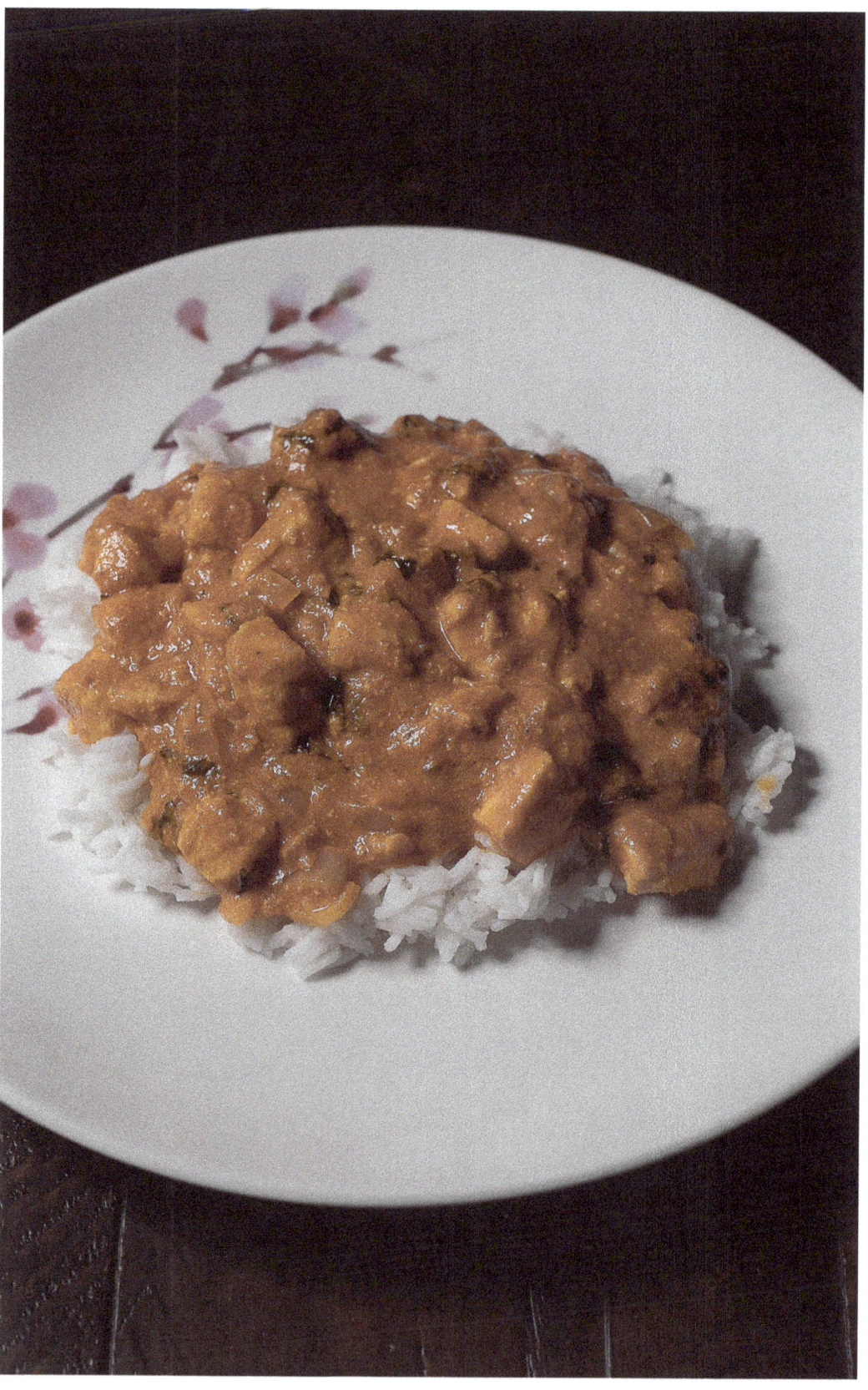

# Chicken Tikka Masala

*This dish is also often known as Butter Chicken.*

*Marinade*
1/4 cup plain Greek yogurt
2 Tbsp lemon or lime juice
2 cloves garlic, thinly sliced
1 1/2 pounds boneless, skinless chicken breasts or 6 thighs, diced*

4 Tbsp butter
1 medium yellow onion, finely chopped
black pepper to taste
1 Tbsp fresh ginger, minced
1 1/2 cups canned crushed tomatoes
1 cup heavy cream
1/2 cup fresh cilantro, chopped

*Spices*
1 Tbsp coriander
1 1/2 tsp cumin
1 1/2 tsp paprika
1/2 tsp cardamom
1/2 tsp nutmeg
1/4 tsp cayenne pepper

Combine the yogurt, lemon/lime juice, and garlic in a zipper freezer bag. Add the chicken and toss to coat thoroughly. Seal and refrigerate for at least 1 hour or overnight.

In a small bowl, combine the spices and set aside.

In a large stock pot or Dutch oven melt the butter over medium-low heat. Add the onions and black pepper and sauté until the onions are soft and translucent, but do not brown. Add the minced ginger and sauté until fragrant. Stir in the spices and sauté for 1 minute, then add the tomatoes. Slowly add the cream, stirring constantly. Bring to a boil, then reduce heat to low. Add the chicken*, cover, and simmer on low, stirring frequently, until the sauce thickens, about 1–2 hours. Remove from heat and stir in the chopped cilantro. Serve over basmati rice with warm naan.

*If you use chicken breasts, cook the sauce without it for about 1.5 hours, then put the chicken in for the last 30 minutes.

Makes about 4–6 servings.

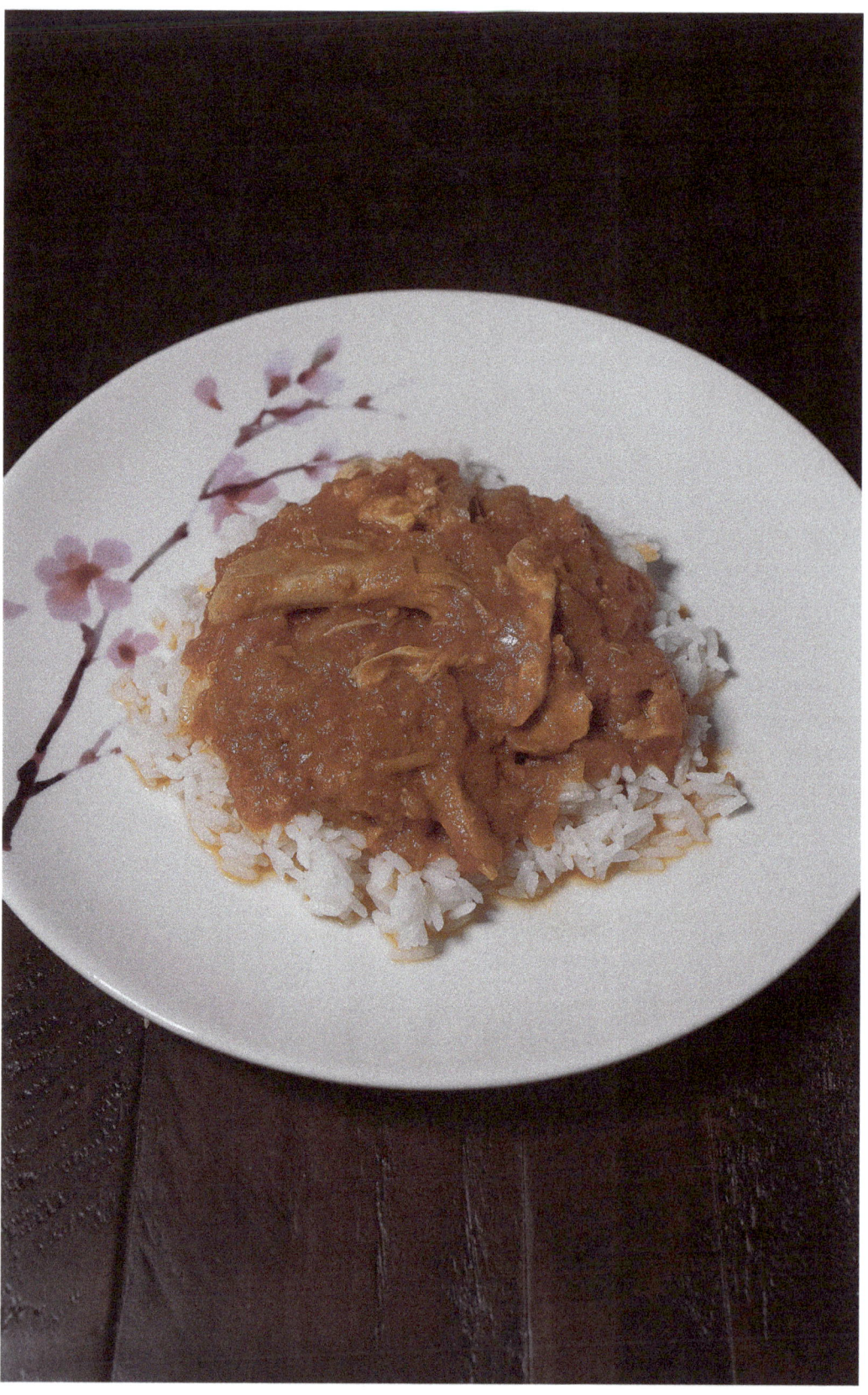

# Doro Wat

*When we lived in Budapest, we frequented a little local café down the block called Kisüzem that always had interesting specials on the menu. One day we smelled something incredibly enticing as the server carried it past us to the next table. We looked at the specials board and saw "Doro Wat" chalked there. We had no idea what it meant, or what was in it, but we couldn't resist that smell. And we were very glad we didn't. This Ethiopian dish relies on a blend of many spices called Berbere, which I was surprised to find in our local supermarket in the US.*

1 Tbsp fresh ginger, peeled and finely minced
2–3 cloves fresh garlic, finely minced
4 small onions, very finely chopped
1 Tbsp Berbere spice blend
1 28-oz can San Marzano tomatoes, hand crushed and fibrous stem ends removed
1/2 cup chicken stock (more if needed to cover chicken)
pinch of sugar
4 chicken thighs, bone-in, skin-on or 6 boneless, skinless thighs

Place the ginger, garlic, and onion in a stock pot or Dutch oven, cover, and sweat over medium-low heat for 90 minutes, stirring occasionally.

Stir the Berbere into the onion mixture and cook for a few minutes until fragrant. Add the tomatoes, chicken stock, and sugar. Bring to a boil, reduce heat to medium, cover, and cook for 5–10 minutes. Add the chicken thighs*, pushing them down to submerge them in the liquid. Cover and simmer on low for at least 2 hours, up to 3 hours. Check it occasionally to be sure it's not sticking to the bottom of the pot.

When the chicken is falling-off-the-bone tender, remove it from the pot and let it cool until you can handle it. Continue to simmer the sauce uncovered until it thickens. Pull the meat from the bones and skin and return the meat to the pot. Serve over jasmine rice.

*If using boneless, skinless chicken thighs, cook the onion and tomato mixture for about 1.5 to 2 hours, then add the chicken and cook for another 45 minutes to 1 hour, until the sauce is thick enough, then serve.

Makes 4–6 servings.

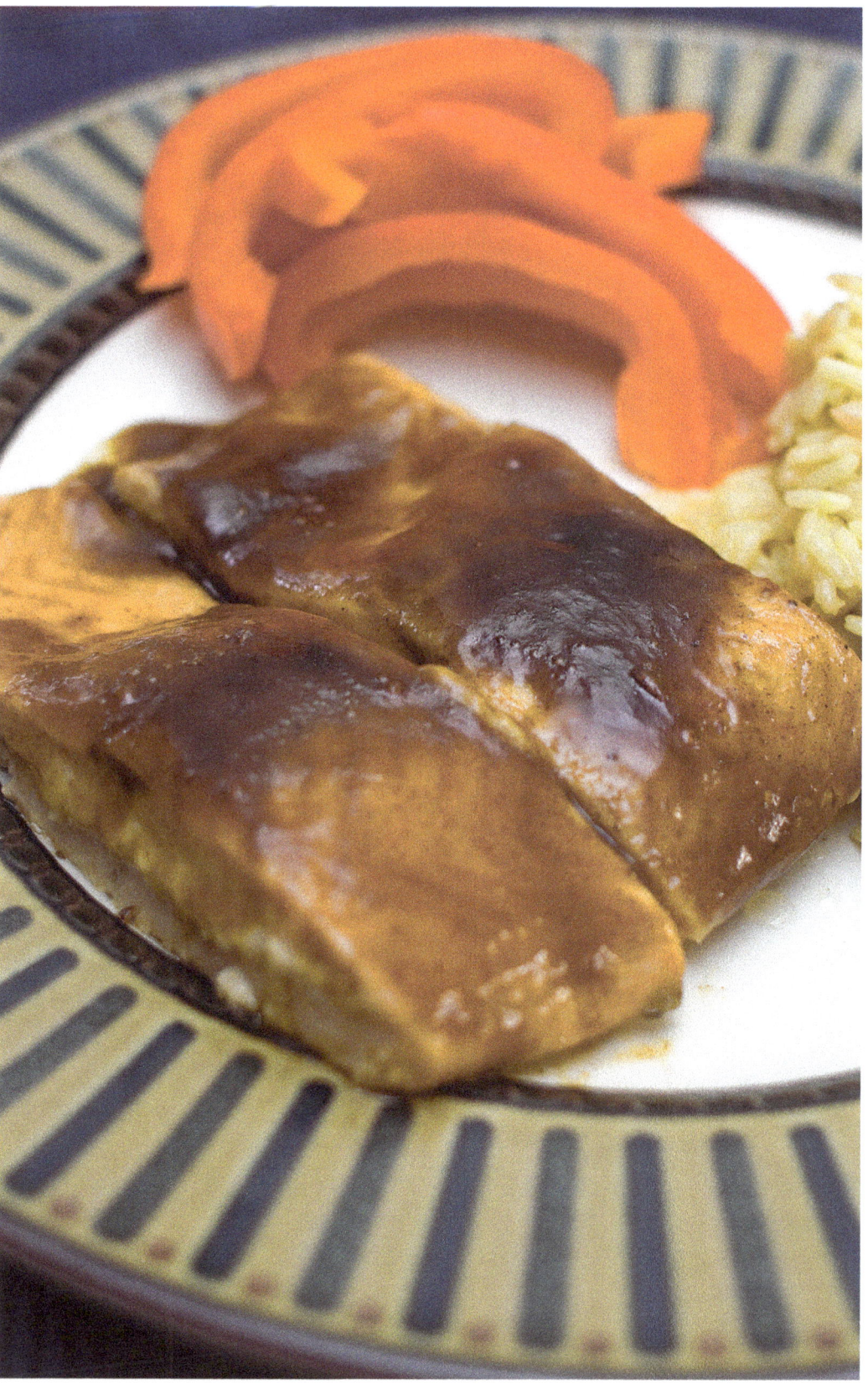

# Glazed Salmon

3/4 cup dry white wine (or water)
1/4 cup butter, cut into small pieces
1 tsp Old Bay seasoning
2–4 large salmon fillets
salt
black pepper
2 Tbsp spicy brown mustard
1/4 cup packed brown sugar

Preheat the oven to 350°F. Bring the wine, butter, and Old Bay to a boil in a small saucepan and boil for 3 minutes. Place the salmon (skin side down, if it has skin) in a deep glass baking dish and sprinkle with salt and pepper. Pour the butter mixture over the salmon. Bake until the salmon is opaque in the center, about 20 minutes. Remove the salmon from the oven and turn on the broiler, moving the rack to the top position.

Mix the mustard and brown sugar until it forms a thick sauce. It should stick to a spoon and drizzle slowly off. Spread the sugar mixture evenly over the salmon, just until it is covered (a thin layer). Broil until the topping begins to bubble, about 1–1 1/2 minutes.

Makes 2–4 servings.

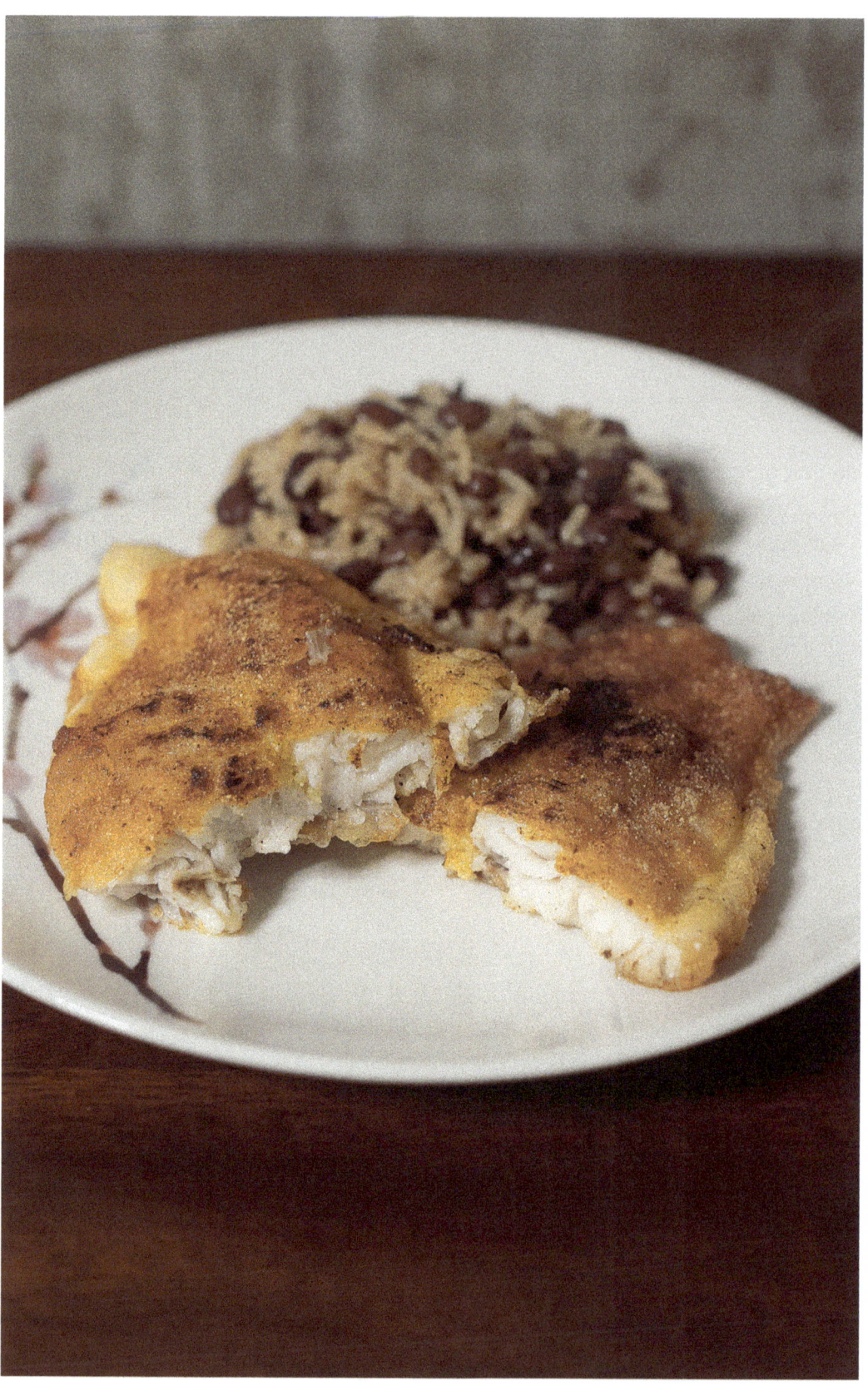

# Pan-fried Catfish

vegetable oil
1/4 cup cornmeal
1/4 cup gluten-free flour*
1/2 tsp salt
1/4 tsp black pepper
2–4 catfish fillets

Pour enough oil in a large cast iron skillet to completely cover the bottom and heat it over medium heat until it shimmers (but not until it smokes).

Combine the cornmeal, flour, salt, and pepper in a shallow bowl or on a large plate. Rinse the fillets under running water and drain. Pat them dry with paper towels. Dredge the fillets in the cornmeal misture, using your fingers to ensure even coverage of the breading all over the fillets. Carefully place the fillets in the skillet and fry for about 7 minutes per side, until golden brown and fish is cooked through and flaky. Do not touch them until you are ready to turn them or the breading will begin to come off.

Serve with *Black Beans and Rice* (7).

*This recipe was tested with a gluten-free baking flour blend of white rice flour, brown rice flour, potato starch, tapioca flour, and xanthan gum.

Makes 2–4 servings.

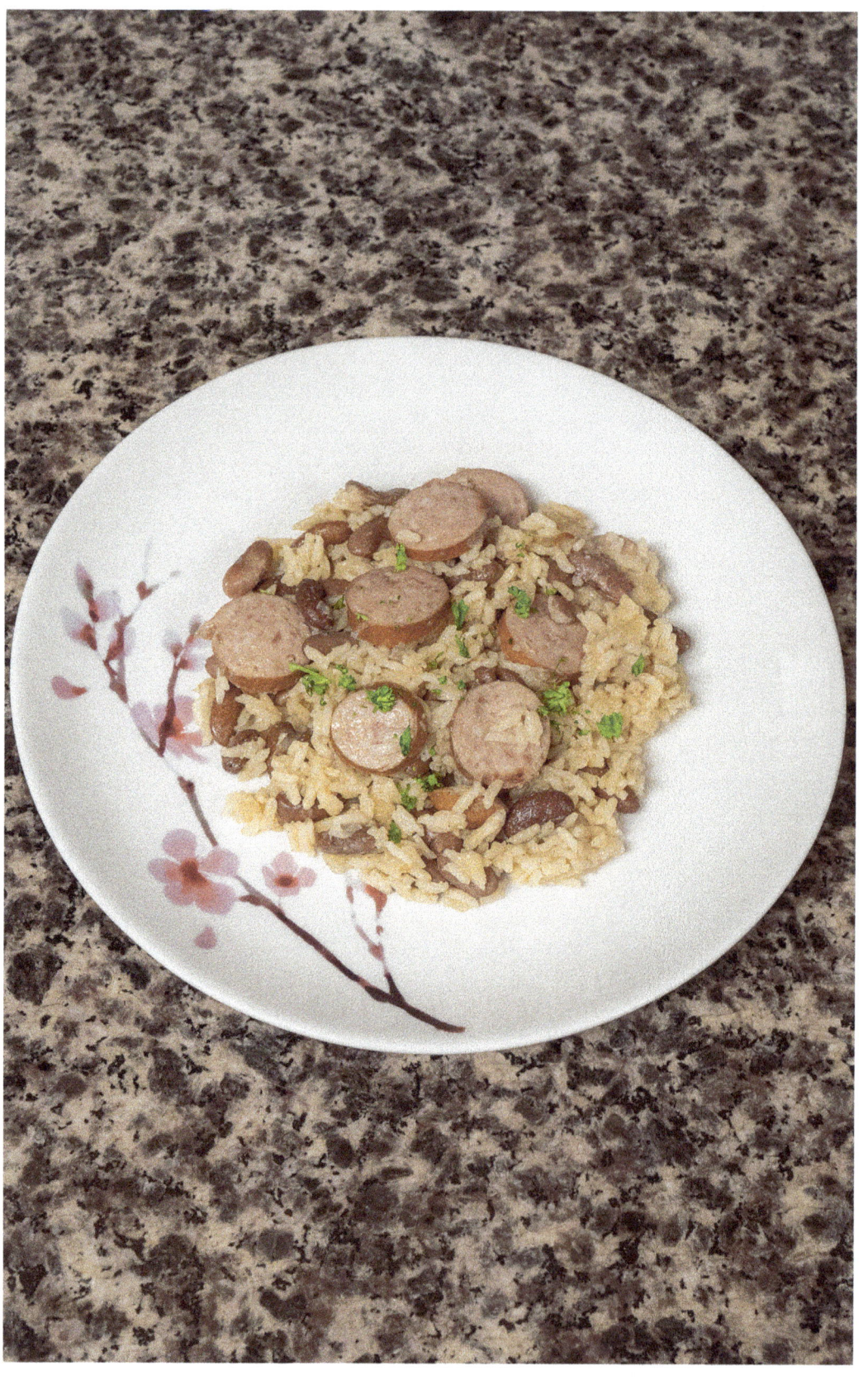

# Red Beans and Rice

1 Tbsp vegetable oil
1 small-medium onion, chopped
2 cloves garlic, minced
1 package gluten-free kielbasa or smoked sausage (13–16 oz), sliced
1 tsp cumin
1/4 tsp chili
1/4 tsp cayenne pepper
1/2 tsp salt*
2 15-oz cans red beans, rinsed and drained (or 1 cup dried beans, soaked, boiled, and drained)
1/2 cup chicken stock or 1/2 cup water + 1 chicken bouillon cube
2 cups water
1 cup white rice

In a large skillet, heat the oil over medium-low heat and sauté the onion and garlic until the onions begin to soften and turn translucent. Add the sausage, turn the heat to medium, and sauté until the sausage begins to brown. Stir in the cumin, chili, and cayenne (and salt, if using) and sauté for about 1 minute until fragrant. Stir in the beans, chicken stock, and water and bring to a boil over high heat. Reduce heat to low, stir in the rice, cover, and simmer 15–20 minutes or until the rice is cooked and all of the water is absorbed. Remove from heat and let stand, covered, for 5 minutes before serving.

*If using dried beans. If using canned beans, omit salt. If you use a chicken bouillon cube, you also may want to omit the salt.

Makes about 4 servings.

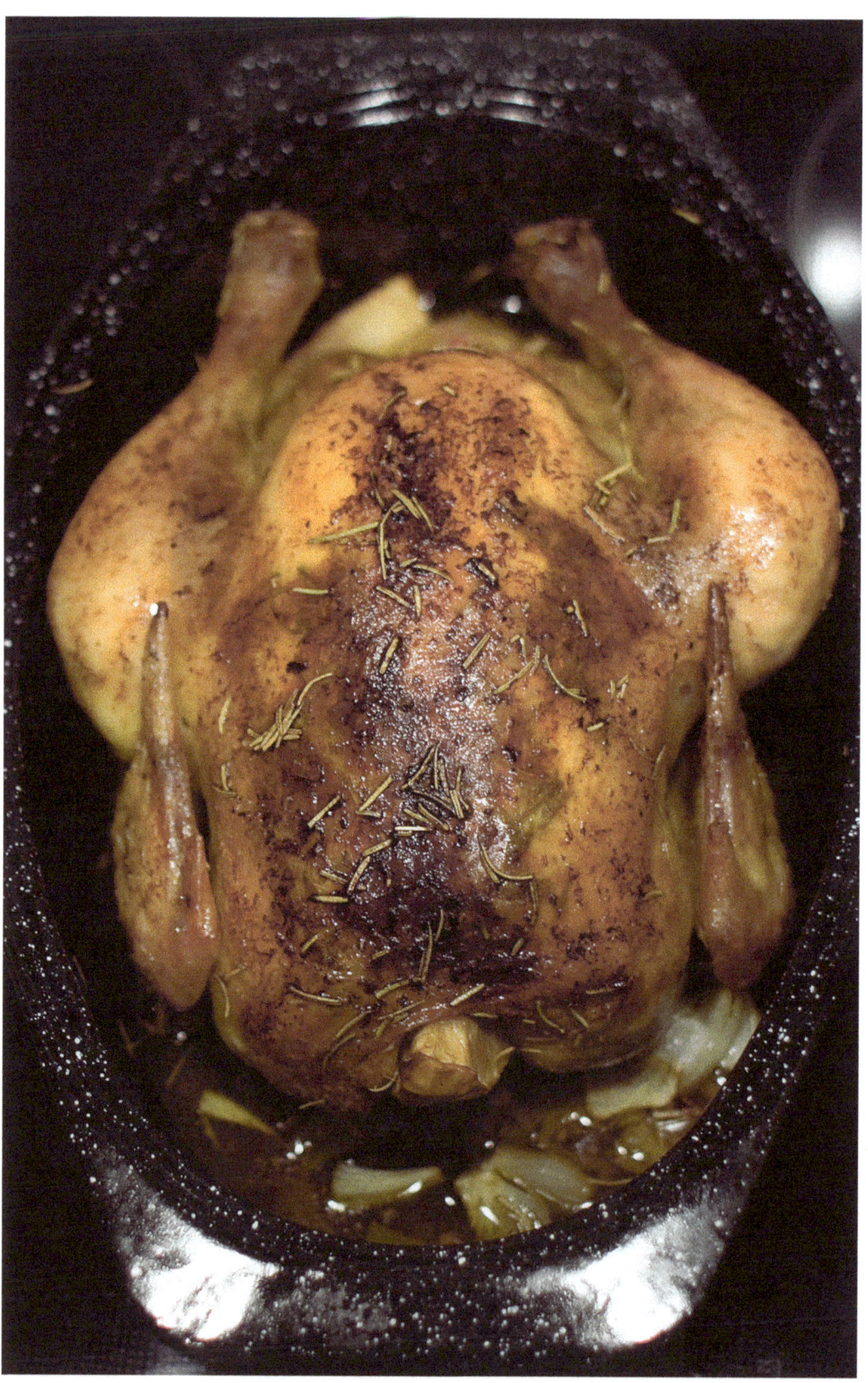

# Rosemary Roast Chicken

4 Tbsp (1/2 stick) butter, softened
3 tsp fresh rosemary leaves, coarsely chopped (or 2 tsp dried)
3 tsp fresh thyme, coarsely chopped (or 2 tsp dried)
1 whole roasting chicken, 1 1/2 to 3 1/2 pounds
2–4 whole rosemary sprigs
1 onion, peeled and cut into large chunks
1 apple (any variety), cored and cut into large chunks

Preheat the oven to 350°F. Combine the butter, rosemary, and thyme to form a compound butter.

Remove the giblets from the chicken, if it has them, and place the bird in a roaster pan, breast up. Run your fingers under the skin of the breast to loosen it, then rub half of the compound butter under the skin. Rub the remaining compound butter over the top of the bird, including the legs. Place the onion, apple, and rosemary sprigs inside the cavity. Tie the legs together with baking twine or an oven-safe elastic band to keep the apple and onion inside. Roast*, uncovered, until a meat thermometer inserted in the thigh muscle (not touching the bone) registers 180°F. Baste about every 15 minutes. Discard the onions and apples before serving.

**Note:** Save the bones from your roast chicken. You can use them to make stock, which you can use in other recipes, such as *Doro Wat* (45). Place the bones in a large stock pot, cover with several quarts of water, and boil for at least an hour. Let it cool, strain the bones out, and freeze the stock in ice cube trays. Place enough cubes to equal 1/2 cup in individual zipper bags. The number of cubes needed for 1/2 cup will vary depending on the size of the ice cube tray's compartments.

*At 350°F, roast for 20 minutes per pound plus 15 minutes.

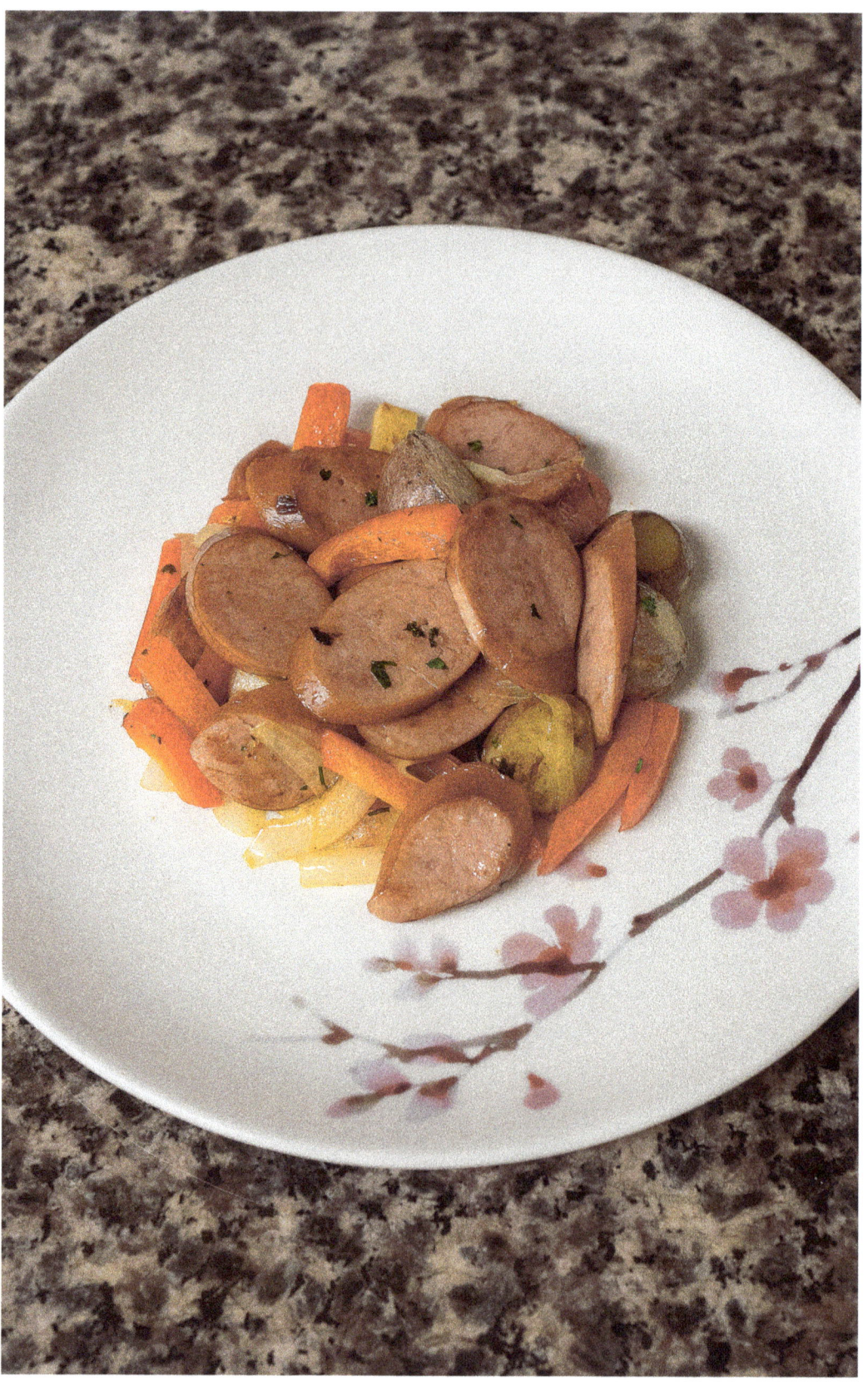

# Sautéed Sausage, Peppers, and Potatoes

*This dish originated on our very first night in Mátészalka, Hungary. As a welcome gift, my fellow teachers had given us salt, bread, onions, and yellow Hungarian peppers. With some Debreceni (a sausage similar to kielbasa) from the Tesco hypermarket down the road, we concocted dinner. It was so tasty, we've kept it in our repertoire, switching to red bell peppers. The* Roasted Potatoes and Shallots *were eventually added because we had some leftover from dinner the night before and weren't sure when else we would use them. They work perfectly in this.*

1 package gluten-free kielbasa or smoked sausage (13–16 oz), sliced
1 medium yellow onion, quartered and sliced
1 red bell pepper, quartered and sliced
leftover *Roasted Potatoes and Shallots* (page 17, optional)

In a medium skillet over medium heat, sauté the kielbasa for about 5 minutes, until they begin to brown. Add the onions and peppers and sauté until the peppers begin to soften, about 5 minutes. If there is not enough liquid in the pan from the vegetables, add about a half a tablespoon of water. Add the *Roasted Potatoes and Shallots*, if desired. Continue to sauté until the potatoes are heated through and the peppers are al dente.

Makes about 4 servings.

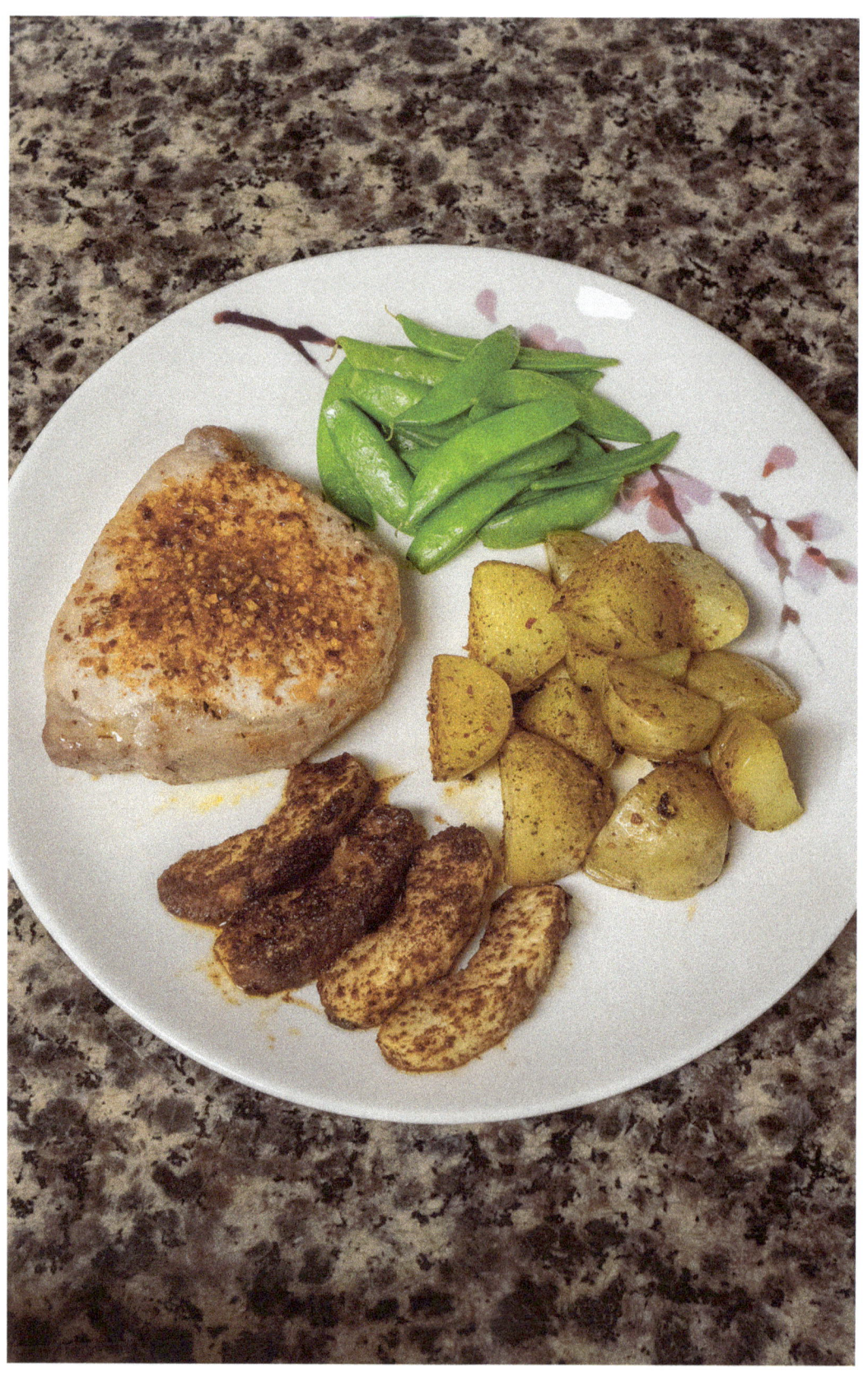

# Sheet Pan Pork Chops

1/4 cup olive oil, divided
1 1/2 pounds mini red or mini gold potatoes, quartered
1/4 tsp salt
1/4 tsp black pepper
southwest seasoning mix
1 large gala or Honeycrisp apple, peeled, cored, and cut into 1/2-inch slices
2 tsp brown sugar
1 tsp ground cinnamon
1/4 tsp ground ginger
4 boneless pork loin chops (1 inch thick and about 6 ounces each)

Preheat oven to 425°F. Line a 15 x 10 x 1" baking pan with foil; brush the foil with 2 teaspoons of olive oil.

In a large bowl, toss the potatoes with 1 tablespoon of olive oil. Place the potatoes in 1 section of the prepared baking pan. Sprinkle the salt, pepper, and southwest seasoning over the potatoes.

In the same bowl, toss the apple slices with 1 teaspoon of olive oil. In a small bowl, mix the brown sugar, cinnamon, and ginger; sprinkle over the apples and toss to coat. Transfer the apples to a second section of the pan.

Brush the pork chops with the remaining olive oil; sprinkle all sides with southwest seasoning. Place the chops in the remaining section of the pan. Bake until a thermometer inserted in the pork reads 145°F and the potatoes and apples are tender, 20–25 minutes. Let stand 5 minutes before serving. Serve with steamed asparagus, green beans, or snap peas.

Makes 4 servings.

# Sheet Pan Tandoori Chicken

*Marinade*

2 Tbsp vegetable oil
4 cloves garlic, minced
2 Tbsp fresh ginger, minced
1 Tbsp chili powder
1 Tbsp garam masala
1 tsp cumin
2 tsp paprika
1 tsp turmeric
1 cup plain Greek yogurt
2 Tbsp lemon or lime juice
2 tsp salt
1/8 tsp black pepper
4 bone-in, skin-on chicken thighs
1 large Yukon Gold potato, cut into 1-inch pieces

*Vegatables*

1 zucchini, cut into 1-inch pieces
1 red bell pepper, cut into 1-inch pieces
1 small yellow onion, halved lengthwise, then sliced into thin half-moons
3 Tbsp vegetable oil
1 tsp cumin
1/2 teaspoon cumin seeds
1/2 tsp salt
1/8 tsp black pepper

*Marinade*

In a small skillet over medium heat, heat the oil. Add the garlic and ginger and cook, stirring constantly, until light brown and fragrant, about 1 minute. Add the chili powder, garam masala, cumin, paprika, and turmeric and cook, stirring constantly, for an additional minute. Set aside to cool.

In a large bowl, combine the yogurt, lemon or lime juice, salt, black pepper, and the cooled spice mixture and stir to combine.

Using a sharp knife, score the skin of each piece of chicken, making two or three shallow cuts about 1 inch apart. Add the chicken and potatoes to the bowl with the spiced yogurt and massage the yogurt into the chicken until all the pieces are well coated. Transfer the chicken, potatoes, and spiced yogurt to a large zip-top freezer bag and set aside for 30 minutes at room temperature, or refrigerate for up to 8 hours.

Set a rack in the upper third of the oven and preheat the oven to 425°F.

*Main Courses*

Remove the marinated chicken from the bag, letting any excess marinade drip off, and arrange the pieces skin side up on a 15 x 10 x 1" baking sheet lined with foil. Scatter the potatoes around the chicken. Roast for 30 minutes, then remove from oven.

*Vegetables*
While the chicken is cooking, place the zucchini, red pepper, and onion in a large bowl. Add the oil, cumin, cumin seeds, salt, and black pepper and mix well.

After the chicken has cooked for 30 minutes, place the vegetables in a single layer in any spaces around the chicken. Return the pan to the oven and roast for an additional 10 minutes. Remove from the oven.

**Optional:** Switch the oven to broil. Return the baking sheet to the oven and broil until the chicken is lightly charred and crispy, 2–3 minutes. Remove from the oven and serve.

Makes 4 servings.

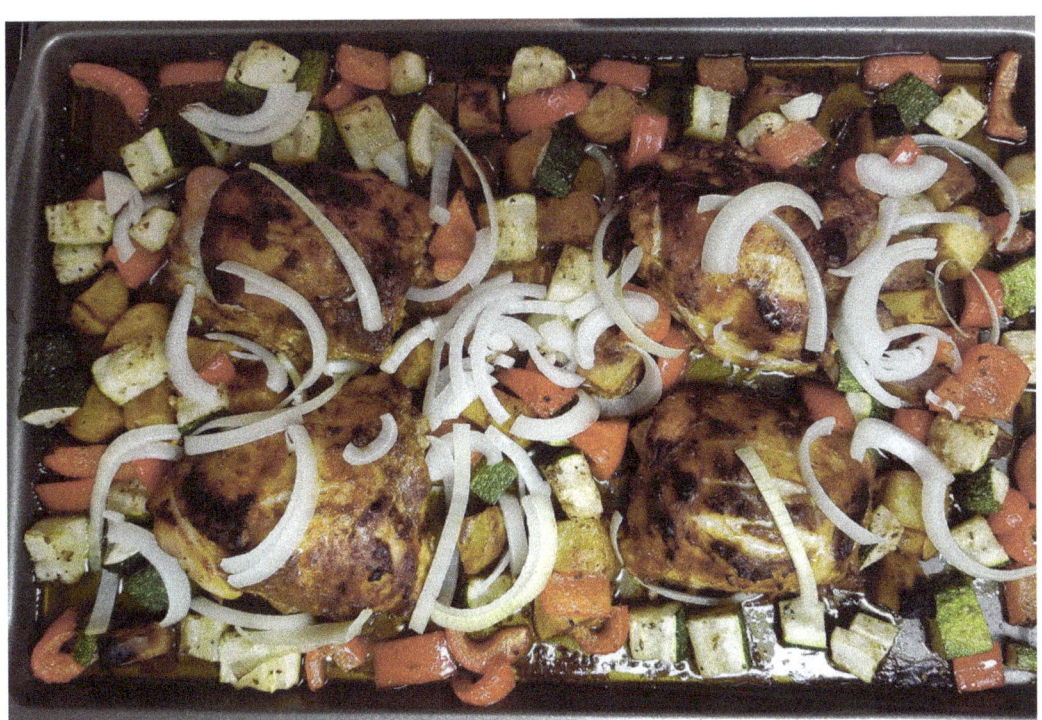

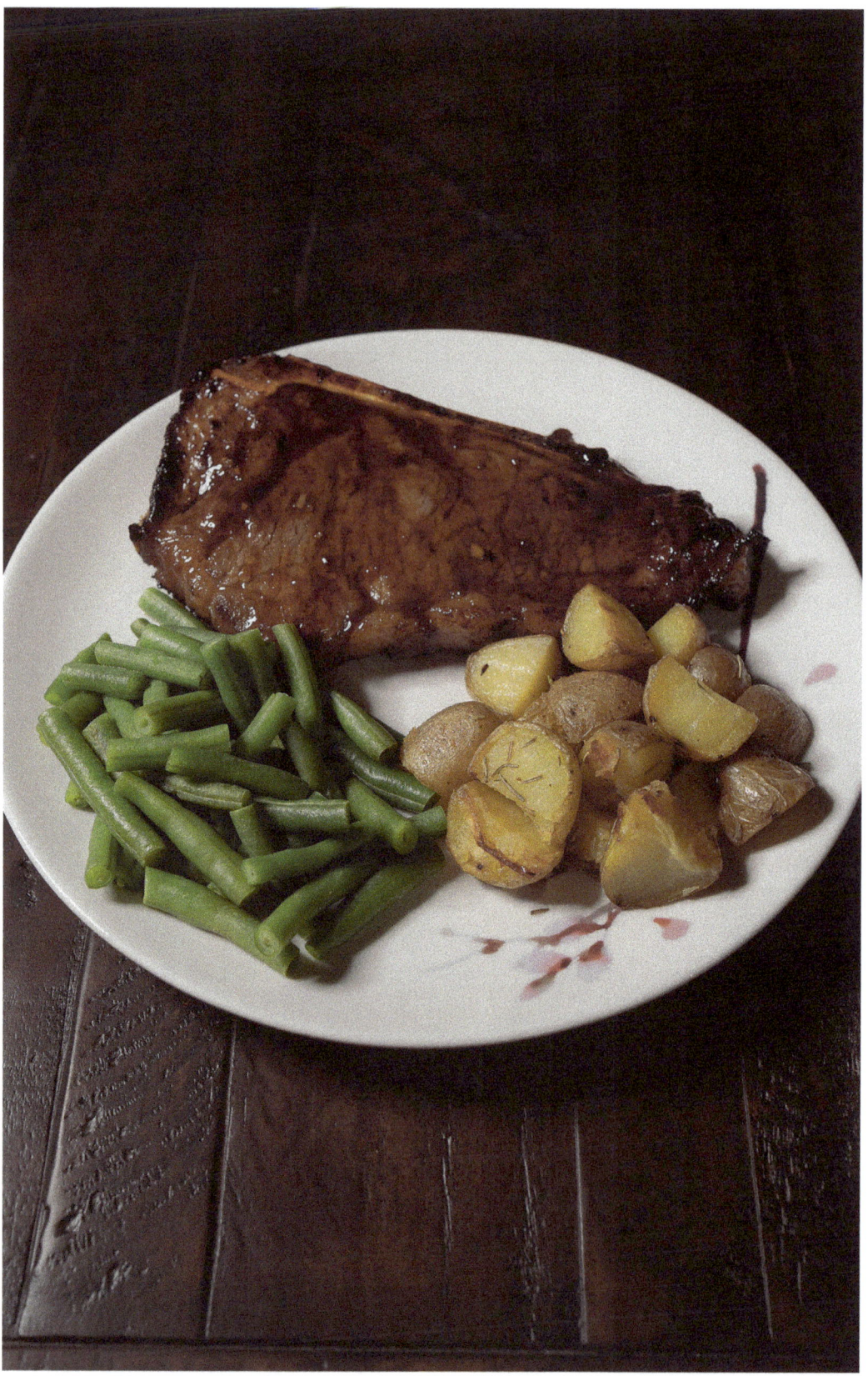

# Steak Maui

*Marinade*

2 cups pineapple juice
1/2 cup low-sodium soy sauce
1/4 cup plus 1 Tbsp apple cider vinegar
2 tsp toasted sesame oil

1/2 cup granulated sugar
2 cloves garlic, finely chopped
1-inch piece ginger, finely chopped

vegetable oil to brush steaks for cooking
2 1" thick bone-in rib-eye or New York strip steaks (about 2–3 pounds total)
1 Tbsp butter for sauce

Combine the liquid ingredients of the marinade and sugar in a small bowl and stir until sugar is completely dissolved. Add garlic and ginger. Transfer marinade to a large resealable plastic bag. Add the steaks and seal bag, pressing out excess air. Chill at least 1 day.

Remove steaks from the bag, reserving 1/2 cup of the marinade. Pat the steaks dry with paper towels and let sit on a cooling rack over a plate until room temperature, about 1 hour.

Place the oven rack 6 inches from the broiler and pre-heat a cast iron skillet on broil for 20 minutes. Brush each steak with oil on both sides and sear in the cast iron under the broiler for 3 minutes per side. Use metal tongs to carefully turn each steak. After the second 3-minute sear, immediately reduce the oven temperature to 500°F and bake the steaks, turning halfway through the cooking time indicated:

| Doneness | 1" thick | 1 1/4" thick | 1 3/4" thick |
| --- | --- | --- | --- |
| Rare (120–130°F) | 0–1 min | 2–3 min | 4–5 min |
| Medium (140–150°F) | 2–3 min | 4–5 min | 6–7 min |
| Medium-Well (150–160°F) | 4–5 min | 6–7 min | 8–9 min |

Remove the steaks to a plate. Let them rest for 10–15 minutes, uncovered. While the steaks are resting, place the skillet on the stove over medium heat. Stir the reserved marinade into the skillet to deglaze it. Add the butter and cook, stirring constantly, until reduced to the desired thickness. Plate the steaks and drizzle the sauce on top. Serve with *Roasted Potatoes and Shallots* (17) or *Rosemary Potatoes* (19).

Makes 2 servings.

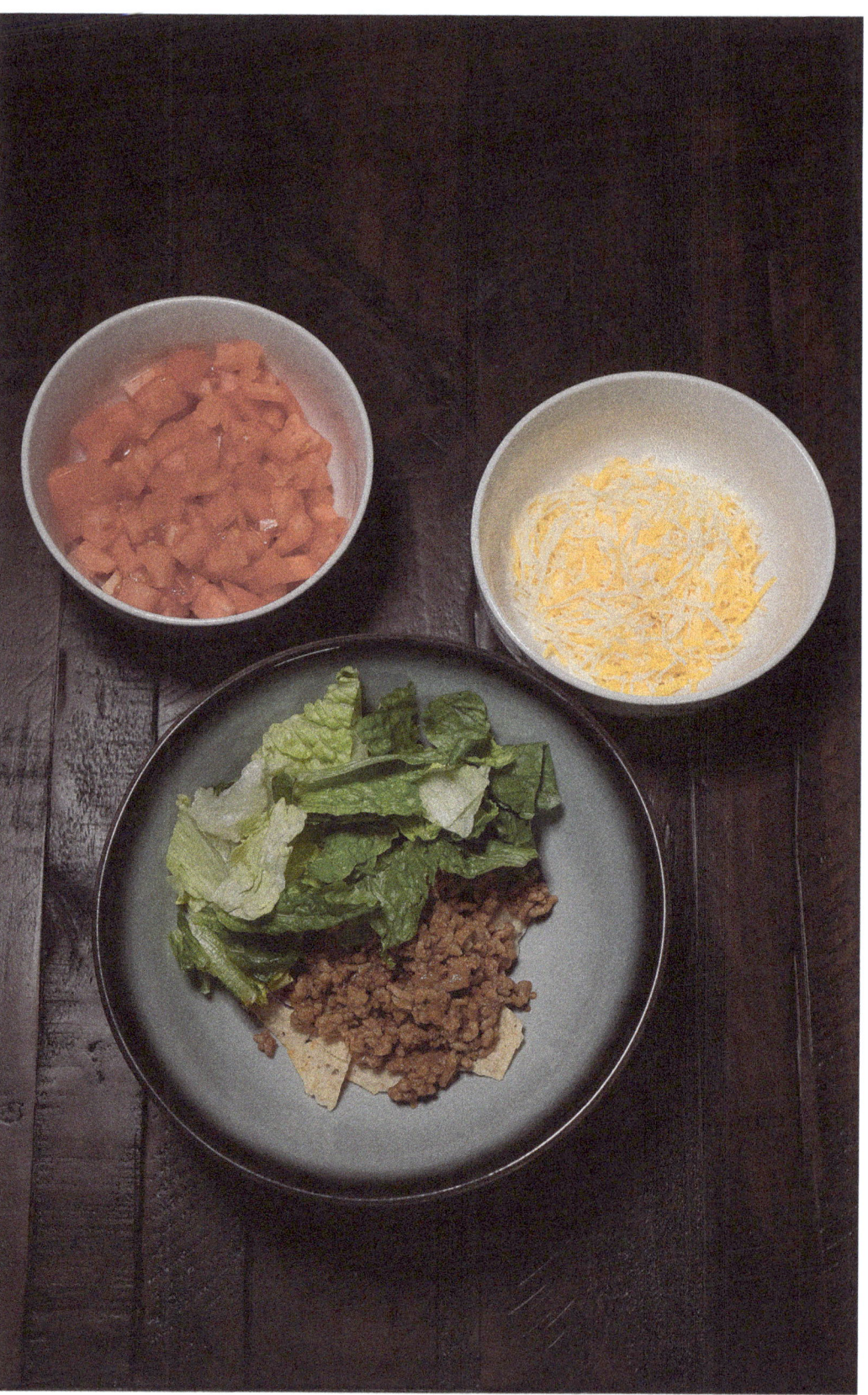

# Taco Salad

1–2 Tbsp vegetable oil
1 medium onion, chopped
2 cloves garlic, minced
1 pound ground beef or pork
1 tsp cumin
3/4 tsp chili pepper
1/2 tsp dried oregano
1/2 tsp paprika
1/4 tsp cayenne pepper
2 Tbsp double-concentrated tomato paste
1/2 cup water
corn tortilla chips
lettuce or bagged salad mix
1 medium tomato, diced
shredded cheese
sour cream
salsa
other toppings

Heat the oil in a medium-sized skillet over medium-low heat and sauté the onion and garlic until just beginning to brown and the onions turn translucent. Add the ground meat, turn the heat to medium, and brown the meat, breaking it up as it cooks. Stir in the spices and sauté for 1 minute, then stir in the tomato paste and water. Bring to a boil, reduce heat to low, and simmer until most of the liquid is gone, stirring occasionally, about 10–20 minutes. Remove from heat.

Crush a handful of tortilla chips in large bowls and spoon the meat over, then top with salad mix, diced tomato, and other toppings.

Makes about 4 servings.

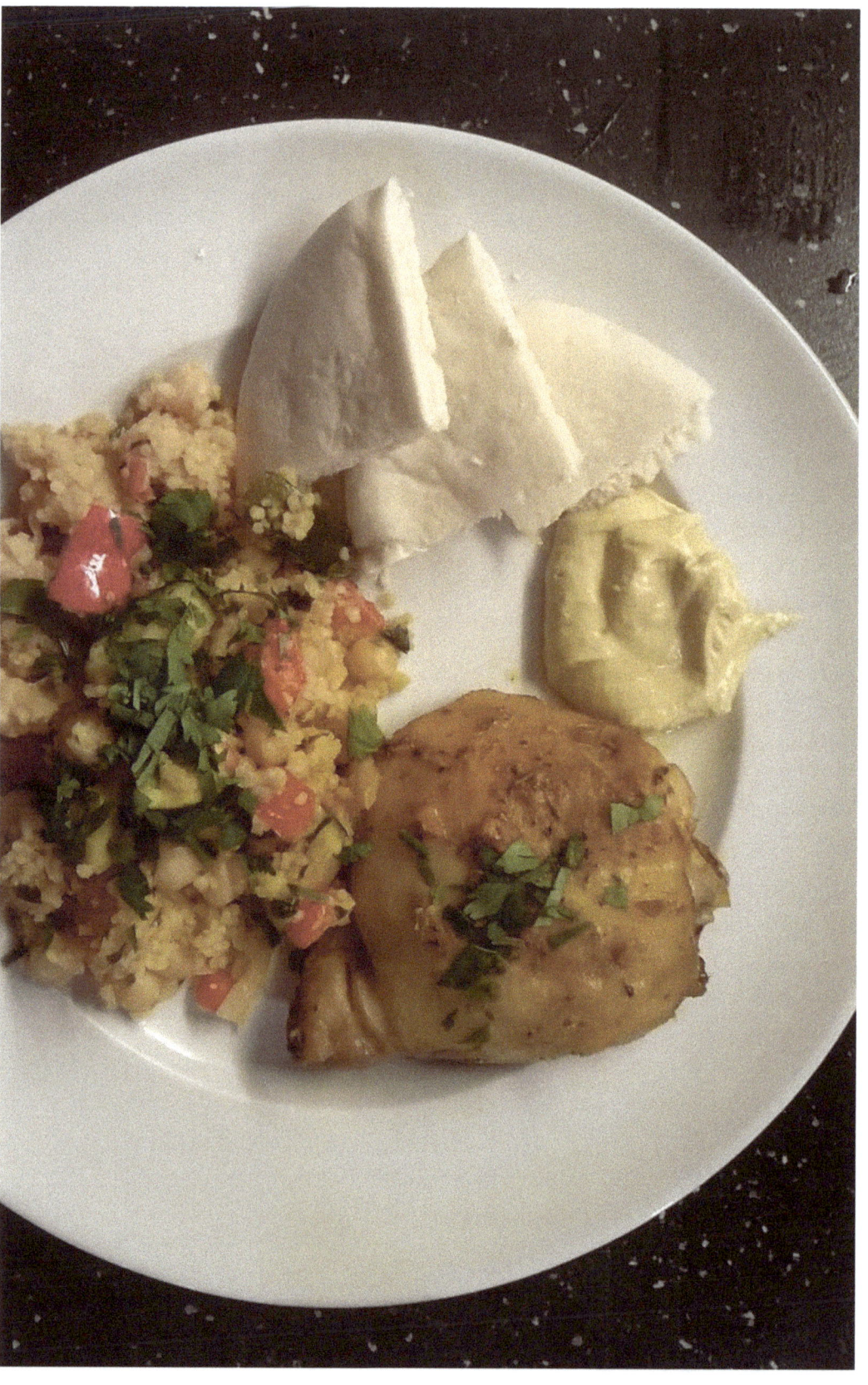

# Turmeric Chicken

2–3 Tbsp olive oil
1 tsp turmeric
1/2 tsp dried oregano
salt to taste
black pepper to taste
2 cloves garlic, roughly chopped
4 bone-in, skin-on chicken thighs
hummus

Combine the oil, spices, and garlic in a plastic bag or container big enough to hold the chicken. Add the chicken and turn each piece several times to coat. Seal the container and place in the refrigerator overnight to marinate.

Preheat oven to 375°F. Place the chicken in a casserole dish, pour the remaining marinade and garlic over it, and bake until the internal temperature is at least 165°F, about 45 minutes.

Serve with hummus as a dipping sauce.

Makes 4 servings.

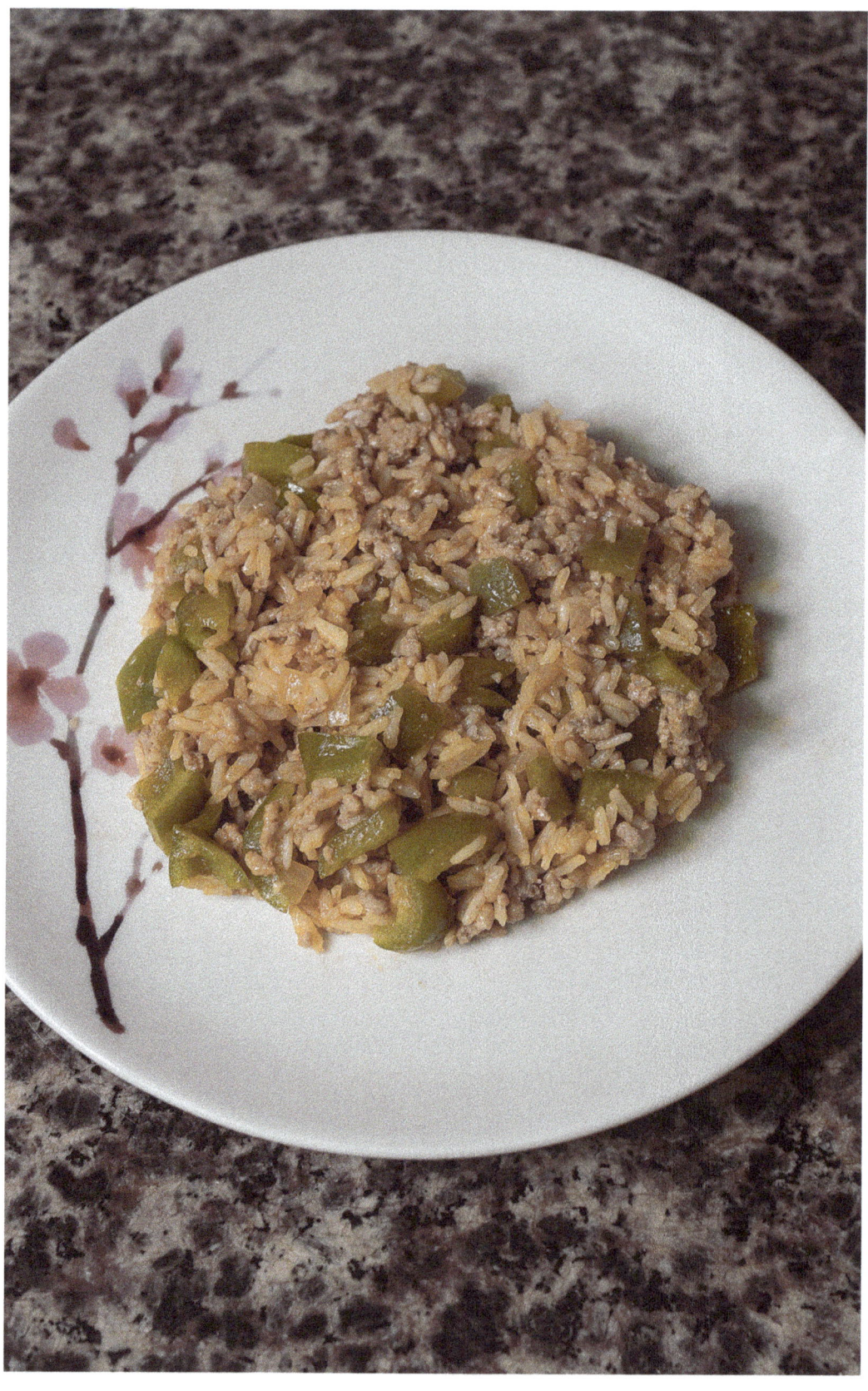

# Unstuffed Peppers

*We love stuffed peppers, but they take some time and effort to make. This one-skillet version tastes every bit as good, but is much faster and easier to put together.*

1 Tbsp vegetable oil
1 medium onion, chopped
2 cloves garlic, minced
1 pound ground beef or pork
1–2 tsp cumin
1/2 tsp dried oregano
1/4 tsp cayenne pepper
1 chicken bouillon cube
2 1/4 cups water
1 cup white rice
2 large green bell peppers, chopped
2 Tbsp double-concentrated tomato paste
shredded mozzarella

Heat the oil in a large skillet over medium-low heat and sauté the onion and garlic until the onions begin to soften and turn translucent. Add the ground meat and sauté until the meat is cooked, breaking it up as it cooks. Stir in the cumin, oregano, cayenne, and bouillon cube and sauté for one minute, breaking up the bouillon cube. Stir in the water, rice, green pepper, and tomato paste. Bring to a boil, stir, reduce heat to low, cover, and simmer 20–25 minutes or until the water is absorbed and the rice is fully cooked. Serve topped with mozzarella.

Makes about 4 servings.

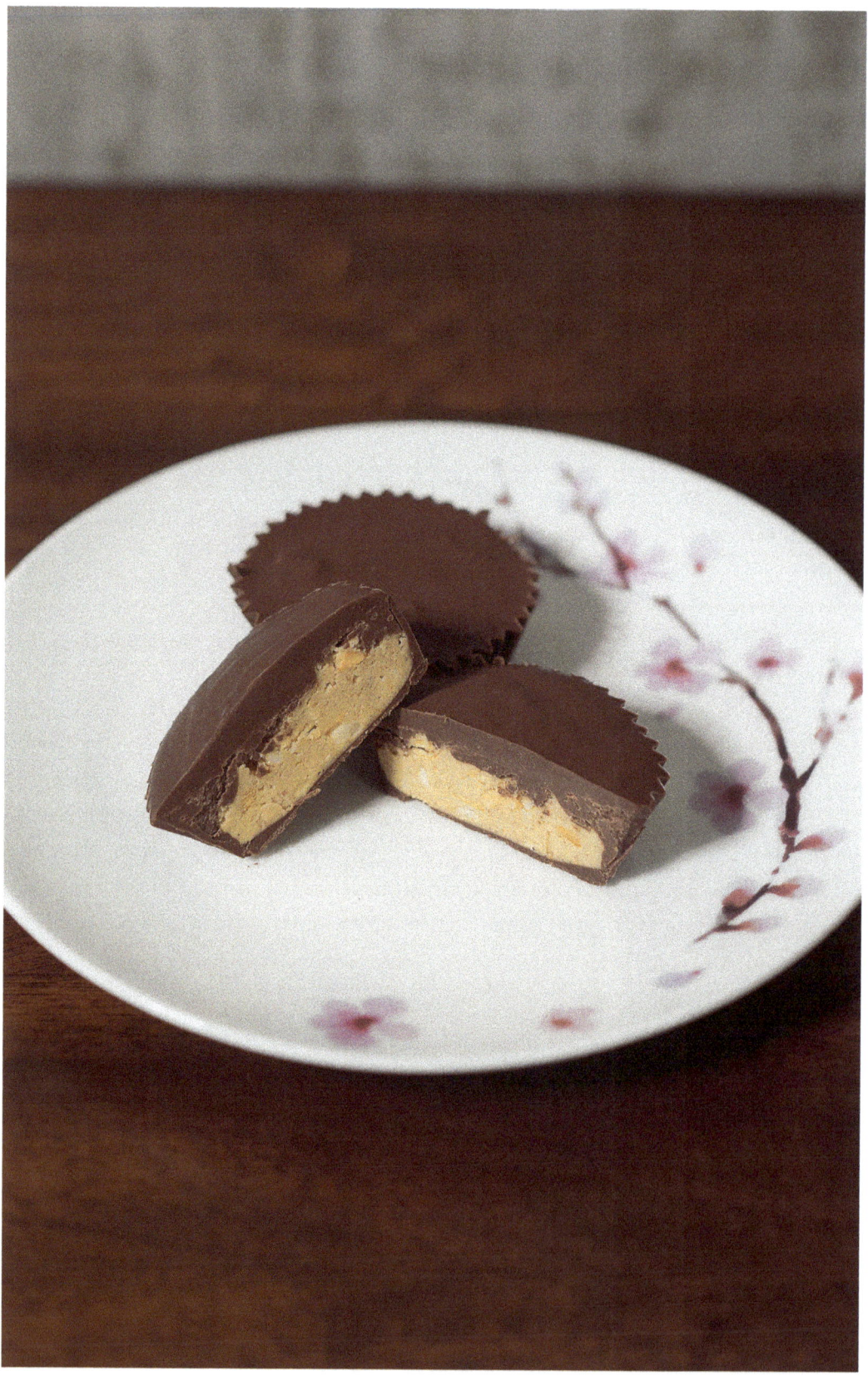

# Desserts

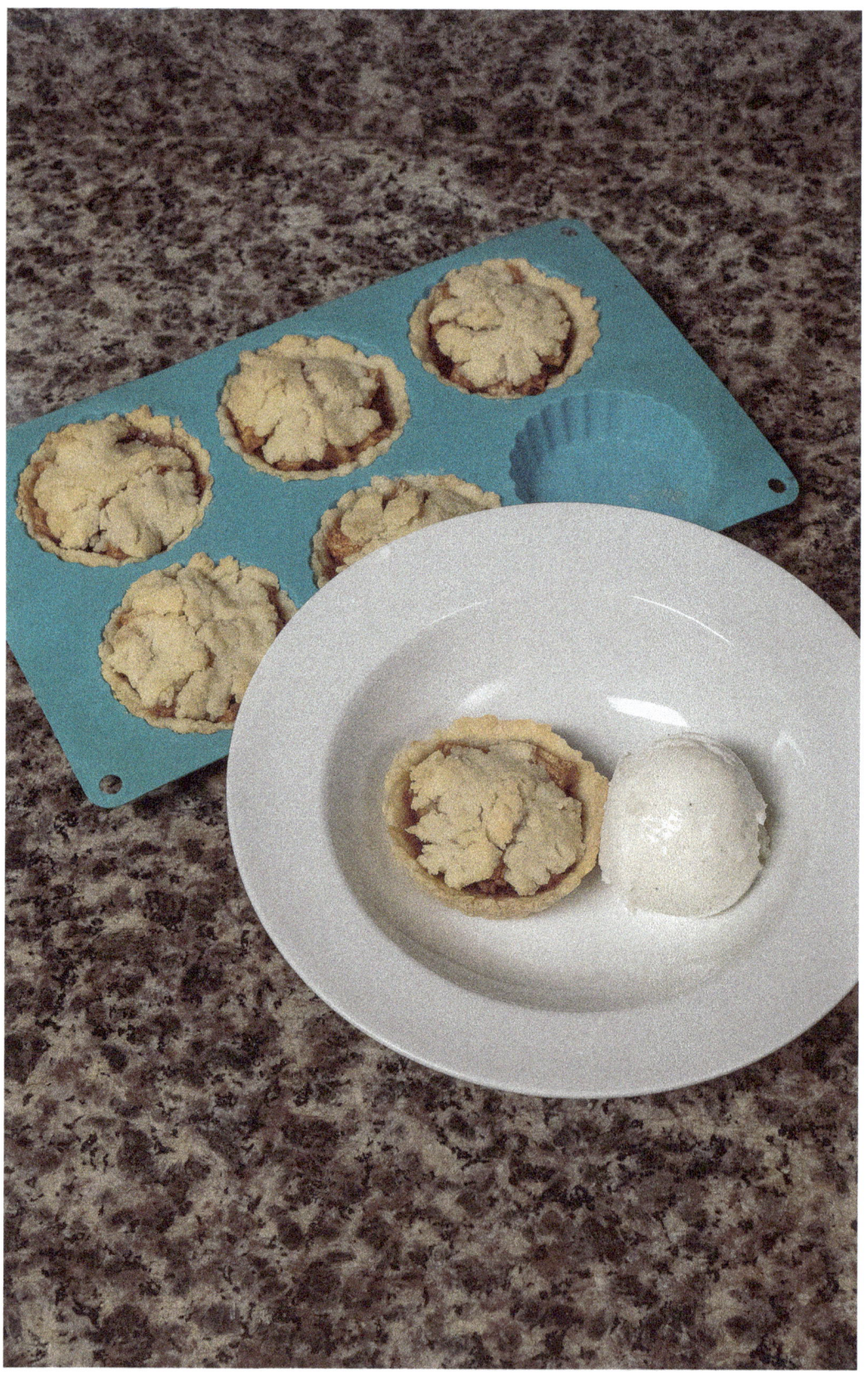

# Apple Tartlets

*French tart pastry*
6 Tbsp butter, cut into pieces
1 Tbsp granulated sugar
1 Tbsp vegetable oil
3 Tbsp water
1 cup plus 1 Tbsp gluten-free flour*

*Filling*
1 large apple (or 2 small/medium)
1 tsp lemon juice
1/4 cup granulated sugar
1 tsp cinnamon
dash of salt

Preheat oven to 400°F. In a medium-sized glass casserole pan with a lid, combine the butter, sugar, oil, and water. Place the covered casserole in the oven for 15 minutes, or until the butter is bubbling and starts to brown just around the edges. Carefully remove from the oven and add the flour, quickly stirring (may splatter) until it comes together and forms a ball that pulls away from the sides of the dish. When the dough is cool enough to handle, divide 2/3 of it between 6 oven-safe silicone mini tart cups (see photo opposite) and press the dough evenly across the bottom and up the sides. You will need to work fairly quickly before it cools too much as it will start to crumble.

Peel, core, and dice the apple and mix in the remaining ingredients. Divide the apple between the tartlets. Divide the remaining pastry dough into 6 equal portions, flatten each carefully with your fingers, and place over the filling. It should not completely cover the filling and can also be crumbled over the top. Bake at 400°F for 30 minutes. Allow to cool, then carefully pop each tartlet out of the silicone mold to serve.

*This recipe was tested with a gluten-free baking flour blend of white rice flour, brown rice flour, potato starch, tapioca flour, and xanthan gum.

Makes 6 tartlets.

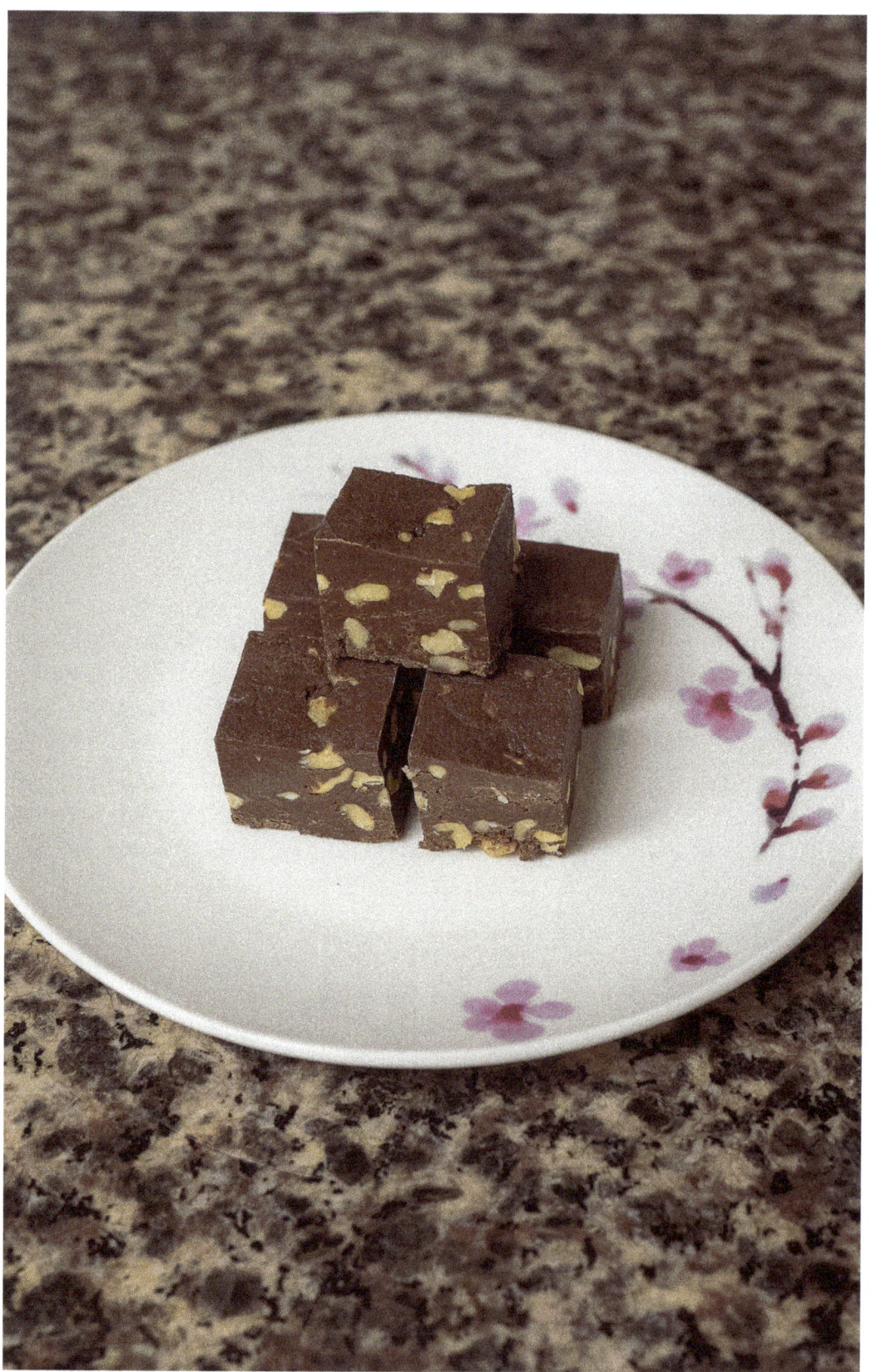

# Easy Fudge

2 12-oz bags semi-sweet chocolate chips
1 14-oz can sweetened condensed milk
1 1/2 tsp vanilla extract
1 cup chopped walnuts

In a heavy saucepan over low heat, melt the chips and condensed milk, stirring occasionally, until smooth. Remove from heat and stir in the vanilla and nuts. Spread evenly into a waxed paper–lined 8- or 9-inch square pan. Chill for at least 2 hours, until firm, then turn onto a cutting board, peel off the waxed paper, and cut into squares. Store in a sealed container in the refrigerator or freezer.

Makes 36–49 squares.

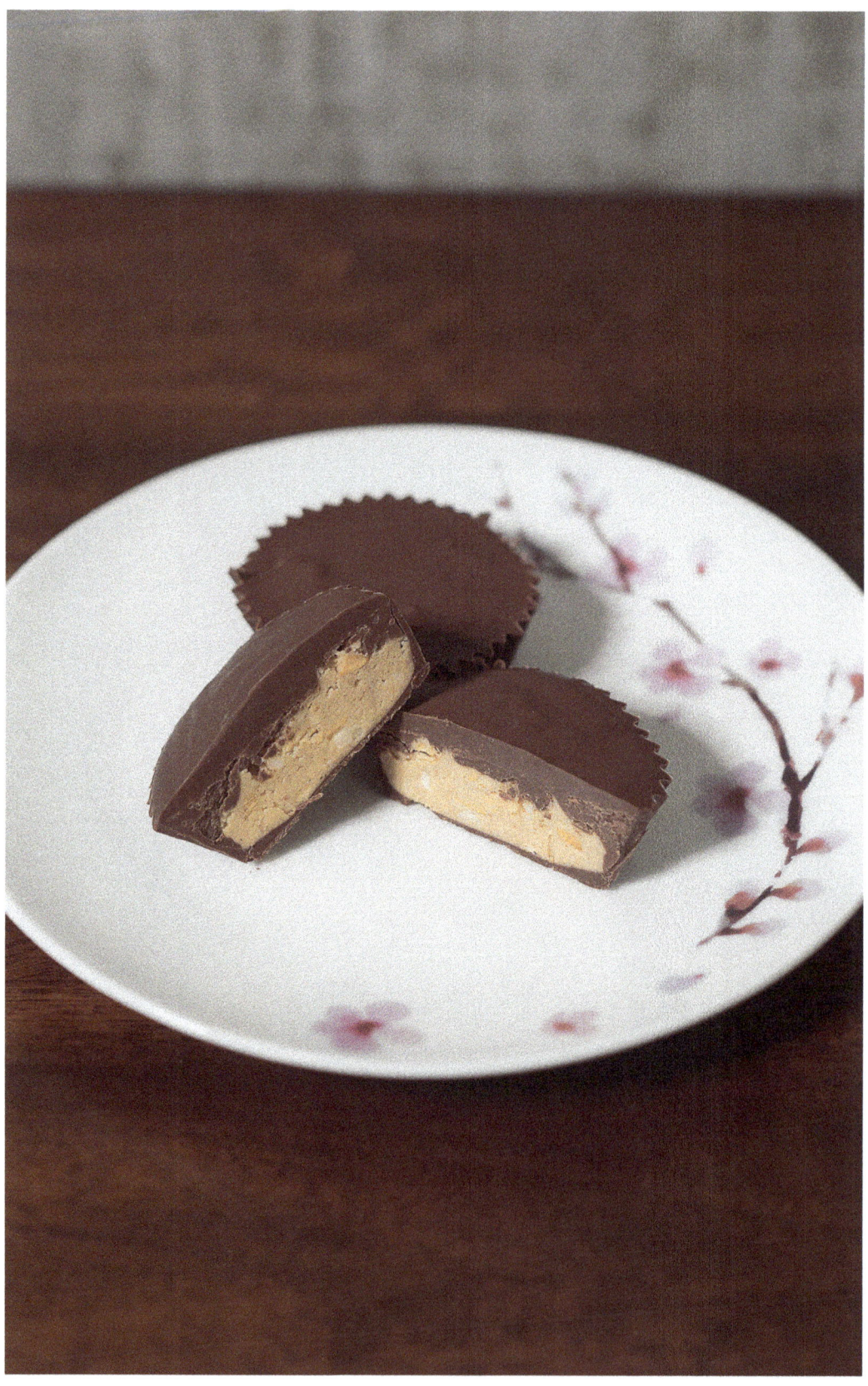

# Peanut Butter Cups

1/2 cup butter (1 stick), softened
1 tsp vanilla extract
16-oz jar extra crunchy peanut butter
1 1/2 to 2 cups powdered sugar (to taste)
3 cups semi-sweet chocolate chips
1/2 cup shortening
24 paper or foil muffin cups

Cream together the butter and vanilla extract, then stir in the peanut butter until fully combined. Mix in the powdered sugar a half a cup at a time (to taste) until fully combined. Set aside.

Melt the chocolate chips and shortening in a double boiler, or in a stainless steel bowl placed over a saucepan of simmering water, stirring until completely smooth. Spoon about 1–2 teaspoons of melted chocolate into 24 muffin cups and roll each around carefully to coat the bottom and halfway up the sides. Place on a baking sheet and refrigerate to set, about 10–15 minutes.

Press a large tablespoon of the peanut butter mixture into each chocolate-lined muffin cup, leaving a small amount of space around the sides and making the top fairly level. Pour melted chocolate over the top, enough to cover the top and fill the sides. Refrigerate to set, at least 30 minutes. Store in a covered container in the refrigerator or freezer.

Makes 2 dozen peanut butter cups.

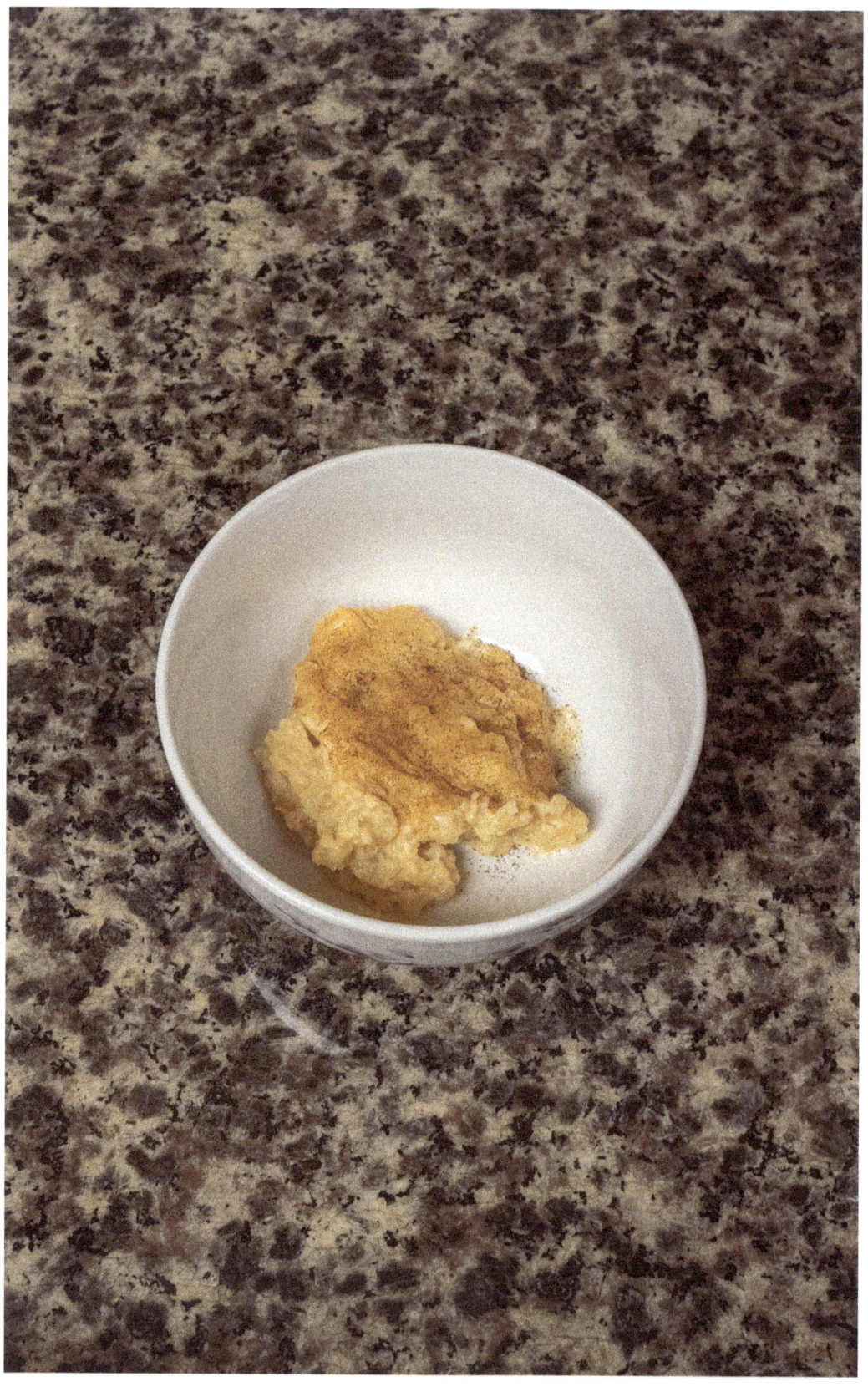

# Rice Pudding

butter for greasing pan
3 1/2 cups milk
1/2 cup uncooked white rice
1/3 cup granulated sugar
1/2 tsp salt
1 tsp vanilla
cinnamon

Preheat oven to 325°F. Grease the bottom and sides of a deep 1 1/2-quart glass baking dish with butter. Set aside.

In a medium saucepan, combine the milk, rice, sugar, and salt. Bring to a boil over medium heat, stirring constantly to keep the milk from scalding. Pour into the buttered baking dish. Cover with foil and bake for 45 minutes, stirring every 15 minutes. Stir in the vanilla, re-cover, and bake for 15 more minutes. Sprinkle with cinnamon before serving.

Makes about 8–12 servings.

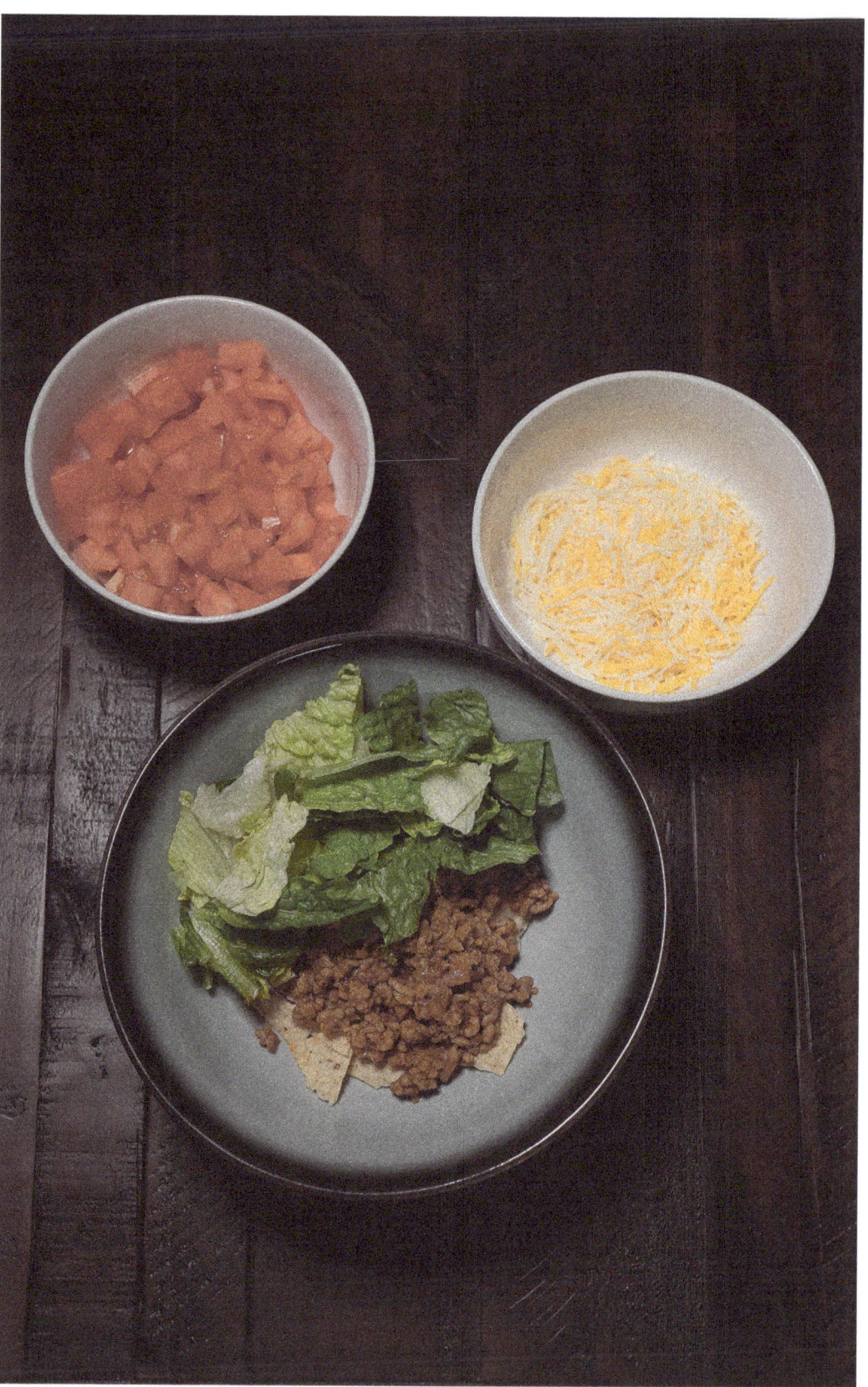

# Index

# Index

**A**

aioli
   Patatas Bravas 15
apple
   Apple Tartlets 71
   Rosemary Roast Chicken 53
   Sheet Pan Pork Chops 57

**B**

bacon
   Corn Chowder 25
   Loaded Baked Potato Soup 27
baked
   Apple Tartlets 71
   Cornbread 9
   Glazed Salmon 47
   Rice Pudding 77
   Roasted Potatoes and Shallots 17
   Rosemary Roast Chicken 53
   Rosemary Potatoes 19
   Sheet Pan Pork Chops 57
   Sheet Pan Tandoori Chicken 58
   Steak Maui 61
   Turmeric Chicken 65
basil
   Broiled Tilapia 37
bay leaf
   Hungarian Pickled Cabbage 11
   Pot au Feu 31
beans
   black and rice 7
   butter, canned
      White Chicken Chili 33
   canned
      Black Beans and Rice 7
      Chili 23
      Red Beans and Rice 51
      White Chicken Chili 33
   Chili 23
   dried
      Black Beans and Rice 7
      Chili 23
   how to use 1
   Red Beans and Rice 51
   great northern, canned
      White Chicken Chili 33
   red and rice 51
beef
   ground
      Chili 23
      Picadillo 29
      Taco Salad 63
      Unstuffed Peppers 67
   short ribs
      Pot au Feu 31
   Steak Maui 61
   stewing
      Pot au Feu 31
   stock
      Picadillo 29
      Pot au Feu 31
berbere spice blend 45
Black Beans and Rice 7, 49
bouillon cube, chicken
   Caribbean Chicken, Chorizo, and Rice 39
   Red Beans and Rice 51
   Unstuffed Peppers 67
bouquet garni
   Pot au Feu 2, 31
broiled
   Glazed Salmon 47
   Steak Maui 61
   tilapia 37
broth
   beef
      Picadillo 29
   chicken
      Loaded Baked Potato Soup 27
      White Chicken Chili 33
butter
   Apple Tartlets 71
   Broiled Tilapia 37
   Butter Chicken 43

# Index

Chicken Piccata 41
Chicken Tikka Masala 43
compound
    Broiled Tilapia 37
    Glazed Salmon 47
    Peanut Butter Cups 75
    Pot au Feu 31
    Rice Pudding 77
    Rosemary Roast Chicken 53

## C

cabbage
    Hungarian Pickled Cabbage 11
    Pot au Feu 31
capers
    Chicken Piccata 41
    Picadillo 29
cardamom, ground
    Chicken Tikka Masala 43
carrot
    Pot au Feu 31
catfish, pan-fried 49
cayenne, ground
    Black Beans and Rice 7
    Caribbean Chicken, Chorizo, and Rice 39
    Chicken Tikka Masala 43
    Chili 23
    Marinated Camembert 13
    Picadillo 29
    Red Beans and Rice 51
    Taco Salad 63
    Unstuffed Peppers 67
celeriac
    Pot au Feu 31
celery
    Corn Chowder 25
cheese
    Brie, marinated 13
    Camembert, marinated 13
    grated
        Loaded Baked Potato Soup 27
    Hermelin, marinated 13

mozzarella
    Unstuffed Peppers 67
shredded
    Taco Salad 63
    Unstuffed Peppers 67
    White Chicken Chili 33
chicken
    boneless, skinless breast
        Caribbean Chicken, Chorizo, and Rice 39
        Chicken Piccata 41
        Chicken Tikka Masala 43
        White Chicken Chili 33
    Butter Chicken 43
    tenders
        White Chicken Chili 33
    thighs
        bone-in, skin-on
            Doro Wat 45
            Sheet Pan Tandoori Chicken 58
            Turmeric Chicken 65
        boneless, skinless
            Chicken Tikka Masala 43
            Doro Wat 45
    whole roasting
        Rosemary Roast Chicken 53
chili, ground
    Chili 23
    Red Beans and Rice 51
    Sheet Pan Tandoori Chicken 58
    Taco Salad 63
chips
    chocolate
        Easy Fudge 73
        Peanut Butter Cups 75
    tortilla
        Taco Salad 63
chive
    Loaded Baked Potato Soup 27
chocolate chips
    Easy Fudge 73
    Peanut Butter Cups 75

*81*

# Index

chorizo, Spanish
    Caribbean Chicken, Chorizo, and Rice 39
cilantro
    Chicken Tikka Masala 43
    White Chicken Chili 33
cinnamon
    Apple Tartlets 71
    Rice Pudding 77
    Sheet Pan Pork Chops 57
clove, whole
    Pot au Feu 31
compound butter
    Broiled Tilapia 37
coriander, ground
    Chicken Tikka Masala 43
Cornbread 9
    with Chili 23
corn
    cream-style, canned
        Corn Chowder 25
    whole kernel, canned
        White Chicken Chili 33
cornmeal
    Cornbread 9
    Pan-fried Catfish 49
cornstarch
    Chicken Piccata 41
    Chili 23
    Corn Chowder 25
    Loaded Baked Potato Soup 27
    Pot au Feu 31
    White Chicken Chili 33
cream
    heavy
        Chicken Tikka Masala 43
    sour
        Taco Salad 63
        White Chicken Chili 33
cumin
    ground
        Black Beans and Rice 7
        Caribbean Chicken, Chorizo, and Rice 39
        Chicken Tikka Masala 43
        Chili 23
        Picadillo 29
        Red Beans and Rice 51
        Sheet Pan Tandoori Chicken 58
        Taco Salad 63
        Unstuffed Peppers 67
        White Chicken Chili 33
    seeds
        Sheet Pan Tandoori Chicken 58

## D
Doro Wat 45

## E
egg
    Cornbread 9

## F
fish
    catfish, pan-fried 49
    salmon, glazed 47
    tilapia, broiled 37
flour, gluten-free
    Apple Tartlets 71
    Chicken Piccata 41
    Cornbread 9
    Pan-fried Catfish 49

## G
garam masala
    Sheet Pan Tandoori Chicken 58
garlic
    Black Beans and Rice 7
    Broiled Tilapia 37
    Caribbean Chicken, Chorizo, and Rice 39
    Chicken Tikka Masala 43
    Chili 23
    Doro Wat 45
    Marinated Camembert 13
    Patatas Bravas 15
    Picadillo 29
    Red Beans and Rice 51

Sheet Pan Tandoori Chicken 58
Steak Maui 61
Taco Salad 63
Turmeric Chicken 65
Unstuffed Peppers 67
White Chicken Chili 33

ginger
    fresh
        Chicken Tikka Masala 43
        Doro Wat 45
        how to peel 1
        Sheet Pan Tandoori Chicken 58
        Steak Maui 61
    ground
        Sheet Pan Pork Chops 57

## H

herbs, *see also specific herbs*
    basil
        Broiled Tilapia 37
    bay leaf
        Hungarian Pickled Cabbage 11
        Pot au Feu 31
    bouquet garni
        Pot au Feu 2, 31
    chive
        Loaded Baked Potato Soup 27
    cilantro
        Chicken Tikka Masala 43
        White Chicken Chili 33
    clove, whole
        Pot au Feu 31
    fresh, how to use 1
    oregano
        Caribbean Chicken, Chorizo, and Rice 39
        Turmeric Chicken 65
        Unstuffed Peppers 67
        White Chicken Chili 33
    parsley, fresh
        Pot au Feu 31
        Roasted Potatoes and Shallots 17
        Rosemary Potatoes 19

rosemary
    Pot au Feu 31
    potatoes 19
    roast chicken 53
thyme
    Marinated Camembert 13
    Pot au Feu 31
hummus
    Turmeric Chicken 65

## J

juice
    lemon
        Apple Tartlets 71
        Broiled Tilapia 37
        Chicken Piccata 41
        Chicken Tikka Masala 43
        Sheet Pan Tandoori Chicken 58
    lime
        Chicken Tikka Masala 43
        Sheet Pan Tandoori Chicken 58
        White Chicken Chili 33

## K

kielbasa 51, 55

## L

lemon
    juice
        Apple Tartlets 71
        Broiled Tilapia 37
        Chicken Piccata 41
        Chicken Tikka Masala 43
        Sheet Pan Tandoori Chicken 58
    slice
        Chicken Piccata 41
lettuce
    Taco Salad 63
lime juice
    Chicken Tikka Masala 43
    Sheet Pan Tandoori Chicken 58
    White Chicken Chili 33

## M

## Index

marinated
    Camembert 13
    chicken
        Chicken Tikka Masala 43
        Sheet Pan Tandoori Chicken 58
    Steak Maui 61
mayonnaise, aioli
    Patatas Bravas 15
milk
    regular
        Corn Chowder 25
        Cornbread 9
        Rice Pudding 77
    sweetened condensed
        Easy Fudge 73
mustard, spicy brown
    Glazed Salmon 47

**N**
nutmeg, ground
    Chicken Tikka Masala 43
nuts, *see walnut*

**O**
oil
    olive
        Pot au Feu 31
        Sheet Pan Pork Chops 57
        Turmeric Chicken 65
    vegetable
        Apple Tartlets 71
        Black Beans and Rice 7
        Chicken Piccata 41
        Chili 23
        Cornbread 9
        Marinated Camembert 13
        Pan-fried Catfish 49
        Patatas Bravas 15
        Red Beans and Rice 51
        Sheet Pan Tandoori Chicken 58
        Steak Maui 61
        Taco Salad 63
        Unstuffed Peppers 67
        White Chicken Chili 33
Old Bay seasoning
    Broiled Tilapia 37
    Glazed Salmon 47
onion
    green
        Loaded Baked Potato Soup 27
    sautéed
        Black Beans and Rice 7
        Caribbean Chicken, Chorizo, and Rice 39
        Chicken Tikka Masala 43
        Chili 23
        Corn Chowder 25
        Doro Wat 45
        Loaded Baked Potato Soup 27
        Picadillo 29
        Pot au Feu 31
        Red Beans and Rice 51
        Sautéed Sausage, Peppers, and Potatoes 55
        Taco Salad 63
        Unstuffed Peppers 67
        White Chicken Chili 33
    sliced
        Hungarian Pickled Cabbage 11
        Marinated Camembert 13
        Rosemary Roast Chicken 53
        Sheet Pan Tandoori Chicken 58
oregano
    Caribbean Chicken, Chorizo, and Rice 39
    Turmeric Chicken 65
    Unstuffed Peppers 67
    White Chicken Chili 33

**P**
paprika, ground
    Chicken Tikka Masala 43
    Chili 23
    Marinated Camembert 13
    Patatas Bravas 15
    Sheet Pan Tandoori Chicken 58
    Taco Salad 63

parsley
    Pot au Feu 31
    Roasted Potatoes and Shallots 17
    Rosemary Potatoes 19
parsnip
    Pot au Feu 31
Peanut Butter Cups 75
peas, frozen
    Picadillo 29
pepper
    green bell
        Corn Chowder 25
        Caribbean Chicken, Chorizo, and Rice 39
        Unstuffed Peppers 67
    red bell
        Chili 23
        Corn Chowder 25
        Hungarian Pickled Cabbage 11
        Picadillo 29
        Sautéed Sausage, Peppers, and Potatoes 55
        Sheet Pan Tandoori Chicken 58
        White Chicken Chili 33
pineapple
    diced
        Caribbean Chicken, Chorizo, and Rice 39
    juice
        Steak Maui 61
pork
    chops, sheet pan 57
    ground
        Chili 23
        Picadillo 29
        Taco Salad 63
        Unstuffed Peppers 67
potato
    canned
        Corn Chowder 25
    fried
        Patatas Bravas 15
    gold
        Rosemary Potatoes 19

    Sheet Pan Pork Chops 57
    Sheet Pan Tandoori Chicken 58
    red
        Loaded Baked Potato Soup 27
        Roasted Potatoes and Shallots 17
        Sheet Pan Pork Chops 57
    roasted
        and shallots 17
        rosemary 19

R

rice
    basmati
        Chicken Tikka Masala 43
    jasmine
        Doro Wat 45
    white
        Black Beans and Rice 7
        Caribbean Chicken, Chorizo, and Rice 39
        Red Beans and Rice 51
        Rice Pudding 77
        Unstuffed Peppers 67
Roasted Potatoes and Shallots 17, 55, 61
rosemary
    Pot au Feu 31
    potatoes 19
    roast chicken 53
Rosemary Potatoes 19, 41, 61

S

salad, bagged
    Taco Salad 63
salmon, glazed 47
salsa
    Taco Salad 63
    White Chicken Chili 33
sauce
    aioli, Patatas Bravas 15
sausage
    *see chorizo or kielbasa*
Sautéed Sausage, Peppers, and Potatoes 17, 55
sesame oil, toasted

# Index

Steak Maui 61
shallot
    Roasted Potatoes and Shallots 17
shortening, vegetable
    Peanut Butter Cups 75
smoke, liquid
    Black Beans and Rice 7
sour cream
    Taco Salad 63
    White Chicken Chili 33
southwest seasoning mix
    Sheet Pan Pork Chops 57
soy sauce
    Black Beans and Rice 7
    Steak Maui 61
spices, *see also specific spices*
    berbere spice blend
        Doro Wat 45
    cardamom, ground
        Chicken Tikka Masala 43
    cayenne, ground
        Black Beans and Rice 7
        Caribbean Chicken, Chorizo, and Rice 39
        Chicken Tikka Masala 43
        Chili 23
        Marinated Camembert 13
        Picadillo 29
        Red Beans and Rice 51
        Taco Salad 63
        Unstuffed Peppers 67
    chili, ground
        Chili 23
        Red Beans and Rice 51
        Sheet Pan Tandoori Chicken 58
        Taco Salad 63
    cinnamon, ground
        Apple Tartlets 71
        Rice Pudding 77
        Sheet Pan Pork Chops 57
    clove, whole
        Pot au Feu 31
    coriander, ground
        Chicken Tikka Masala 43
    cumin
        ground
            Black Beans and Rice 7
            Caribbean Chicken, Chorizo, and Rice 39
            Chicken Tikka Masala 43
            Chili 23
            Picadillo 29
            Red Beans and Rice 51
            Sheet Pan Tandoori Chicken 58
            Taco Salad 63
            Unstuffed Peppers 67
            White Chicken Chili 33
        seeds
            Sheet Pan Tandoori Chicken 58
    garam masala
        Sheet Pan Tandoori Chicken 58
    ginger, ground
        Sheet Pan Pork Chops 57
    nutmeg, ground
        Chicken Tikka Masala 43
    Old Bay seasoning
        Broiled Tilapia 37
        Glazed Salmon 47
    paprika, ground
        Chicken Tikka Masala 43
        Chili 23
        Marinated Camembert 13
        Patatas Bravas 15
        Sheet Pan Tandoori Chicken 58
        Taco Salad 63
    southwest seasoning mix
        Sheet Pan Pork Chops 57
    turmeric, ground
        Sheet Pan Tandoori Chicken 58
        Turmeric Chicken 65
Sriracha
    White Chicken Chili 33
Steak Maui 61
stock

*Index*

beef
    Picadillo 29
    Pot au Feu 31
chicken
    Chicken Piccata 41
    Doro Wat 45
    Red Beans and Rice 51
stovetop cooking
    Black Beans and Rice 7
    Carribean Chicken, Chorizo, and Rice 39
    Chicken Piccata 41
    Chicken Tikka Masala 43
    Chili 23
    Corn Chowder 25
    Doro Wat 45
    Easy Fudge 73
    Loaded Baked Potato Soup 27
    Pan-fried Catfish 49
    Patatas Bravas 15
    Peanut Butter Cups 75
    Picadillo 29
    Pot au Feu 31
    Red Beans and Rice 51
    Sautéed Sausage, Peppers, and Potatoes 55
    Taco Salad 63
    Unstuffed Peppers 67
    White Chicken Chili 33
sugar
    brown
        Black Beans and Rice 7
        Glazed Salmon 47
        Sheet Pan Pork Chops 57
    granulated
        Apple Tartlets 71
        Cornbread 9
        Doro Wat 45
        Hungarian Pickled Cabbage 11
        Rice Pudding 77
        Steak Maui 61
    powdered
        Peanut Butter Cups 75

T
tabasco
    White Chicken Chili 33
thyme
    Marinated Camembert 13
    Pot au Feu 31
tilapia fish, broiled 37
tomato
    chopped
        Chili 23
        Taco Salad 63
    crushed, canned
        Chicken Tikka Masala 43
    diced, canned
        Picadillo 29
    paste, double concentrated
        Caribbean Chicken, Chorizo, and Rice 39
        Chili 23
        Taco Salad 63
        Unstuffed Peppers 67
    San Marzano style, canned
        Doro Wat 45
tortilla chips
    Taco Salad 63
turmeric, ground
    Sheet Pan Tandoori Chicken 58
    Turmeric Chicken 65

V
vanilla extract
    Easy Fudge 73
    Peanut Butter Cups 75
    Rice Pudding 77
vinegar
    apple cider
        Hungarian Pickled Cabbage 11
        Steak Maui 61
    white
        Black Beans and Rice 7

W
walnut, chopped

# Index

    Easy Fudge 73
wine
    red
        Pot au Feu 31
    white
        Loaded Baked Potato Soup 27
        Chicken Piccata 41
        Glazed Salmon 47

## Y
yogurt, Greek plain
    Chicken Tikka Masala 43
    Sheet Pan Tandoori Chicken 58

## Z
zucchini
    Sheet Pan Tandoori Chicken 58

www.ingramcontent.com/pod-product-compliance
Lightning Source LLC
Chambersburg PA
CBHW040751020526
44118CB00042B/2863